Speed Trap

Speed Trap

Inside the Biggest Scandal in Olympic History

Charlie Francis

with

Jeff Coplon

ST. MARTIN'S PRESS
NEW YORK

Some of the conversations related in this book took place a number of
years ago and are reconstructed from memory. In each case, I am confident that I have accurately related the substance and content of what
was said, if not the precise words.

—Charlie Francis

Library of Congress Cataloging-in-Publication Data

Francis, Charlie.
    Speed trap : a track coach's explosive account of how the world's
greatest athletes win with drugs / Charlie Francis with Jeff Coplon.
        p.   cm.
    ISBN 0-312-04877-7
    1. Doping in sports.   2. Anabolic steroids.   3. Track and field
athletes—Drug use.   I. Coplon, Jeff.   II. Title.
RC1230.F73   1991
362.29′08′87964—dc20   90-49392
                                                        CIP

First published in Canada by Lester and Orpen Dennys Publishers Ltd.

First U.S. Edition
10 9 8 7 6 5 4 3 2 1

Acknowledgements

Many people were generous with their time and insights in the development of this book. The authors would particularly like to thank Dr. Mauro DiPasquale, Jim Ferstle, Mike Hurst, Anne-Lise Hammer, and Vera Eubanks.

In addition, the authors are grateful to Michael Carlisle of William Morris, the agent who engineered this collaboration and kept the faith; to Kathryn Dean, our alert and fastidious copy editor; to George Witte, our American editor, and to Richard Johnson, our British editor, both of whom sustained rare good cheer in the face of pressing deadlines; and, especially, to Catherine Yolles, our Canadian editor, who went far beyond the call in keeping this project in order and on track.

Contents

Abbreviations

AAA	Amateur Athletic Association (U.K.)
ABC	American Broadcasting Companies (U.S.)
BBC	British Broadcasting Corporation
COA	Canadian Olympic Association
CTFA	Canadian Track and Field Association
EMS	Electronic Muscle Stimulation
IAAF	International Amateur Athletic Association
IMG	International Management Group
IOC	International Olympic Committee
NBC	National Broadcasting Company (U.S.)
NCAA	National Collegiate Athletic Association (U.S.)
NFL	National Football League (U.S.)
OTFA	Ontario Track and Field Association
TAC	The Athletics Congress (U.S.)
UCLA	University of California at Los Angeles
USC	University of Southern California
USOC	United States Olympic Committee

Speed Trap

The Knock at the Door

The knock came at my dormitory door at 7:30 in the morning, rousing me from sleep. It was Monday, September 26, 1988, in Seoul, South Korea—about 42 hours after my life's great moment. On the previous Saturday, Ben Johnson, the sprinter I'd coached for the past 12 years, had won the Olympic gold medal in the 100 metres, breaking his own world record. His time: 9.79 seconds.

My caller was Dave Lyon, a manager for Canada's track and field team. "We've got to get over to the Medical Commission," he told me. "Ben's tested positive."

With those few words our nightmare began. In our sport, a positive drug test was the ultimate horror. It was like a fatal car crash: You knew it could happen at any time, to almost anyone, but you never believed it could happen to you. There were positives at almost every major meet, but I'd never allowed myself to imagine that one of my athletes would be snared, least of all Ben. The track federations had staged drug tests for 20 years, and in all that time no major star had failed one—not officially, at any rate.

I fumbled with my clothes in a daze. All that Ben and I had worked for was in jeopardy. Our futures now hinged on a laboratory analysis—a preliminary finding that Ben's urine sample had contained traces of a drug banned by the International Olympic Committee.

I knew the test could not yet be conclusive. According to IOC rules, all Olympic medallists must provide a urine specimen after their events. The specimens are divided into "A" and "B" samples and are coded by number. The "name list," which correlates each number to a tested athlete, is held by Prince Alexandre de Merode of Belgium, chairman of the IOC's Medical Commission. Only after an "A" sample turns up positive—where Ben's case stood at the moment—is the name list consulted and the athlete and coach called in for questioning.

The stakes would be high this day. If Ben's "B" sample tested positive as well, the finding would be official. Aside from forfeiting his medal, Ben would be suspended from international competition for anywhere from three months to two years, depending on the drug involved. As Dave Lyon and I took the elevator to the Canadian Olympic Association office on our building's ground floor, I felt spinning with confusion. I assumed that Ben had been nailed for an anabolic steroid, but that made no sense to me. For the past three years, some of my sprinters had been using an injectable form of the steroid furazabol, which we referred to as Estragol. I knew that it couldn't be detected, since the IOC's lab equipment hadn't been programmed to identify furazabol's metabolites, the breakdown substances produced in the body. (Months later, an IOC medical commissioner would verify that fact.) Just what was going on here?

At the team office we met Carol Anne Letheren, our team's *chef de mission*, and Dr. William Stanish, our chief medical officer. Carol Anne said she'd been notified of the positive test result at 1:45 that morning but had decided to spare me a sleepless night. She had wandered the Olympic Village streets until dawn, dwelling on how awful it was and wondering what we would do.

At 10:00 A.M. Dr. Stanish, Dave Lyon, and I drove to the IOC's testing lab in downtown Seoul, where we entered a large, spartan room with an oversized conference table. Already seated were two IOC medical commissioners, Arnold Beckett of Britain and

Manfred Donike of West Germany, and Park Jong Sei, the director of the Olympic drug-testing lab in Seoul. "We've got a positive test here," Beckett led off, "but before we tell you what the substance is, can you think of anything that might have caused it?" This was standard procedure; no mitigating explanation would be allowed after a substance was identified, since statements could then be tailored to fit an athlete's alibi. I had nothing to volunteer, and Beckett dropped his bombshell: The metabolites found in Ben's "A" sample belonged not to furazabol, but to its molecular cousin stanozolol, a popular steroid which we'd known the IOC could test for.

I was floored. To my knowledge, Ben had never injected stanozolol. He occasionally used Winstrol, an oral version of the drug, but for no more than a few days at a time, since it tended to make him stiff. He'd always discontinued the tablets at least six weeks before a meet, well beyond the accepted "clearance time"— the number of days required for a given drug to clear an athlete's system and become undetectable.

After seven years of using steroids, Ben knew what he was doing. It was inconceivable to me that he might take stanozolol on his own and jeopardize the most important race of his life. My first instinct was that he had been set up—that someone had spiked one of his drinks, probably before the race, to allow time for the substance to metabolize.

By 11:00 Ben had joined us and we adjourned to the lab itself, where the sealed container with the "B" sample could be opened. He was less upset than I might have expected—a lot less upset than I was. "I knew something was funny—that guy in the testing room must have messed me up," Ben told us. At Beckett's urging, he elaborated. Amid the hoopla that followed his record run, several unauthorized people had milled through the supposedly secure area. Through most of his 90 minutes in the doping control waiting room—a sparsely furnished place with a couch, a television, and a refrigerator stocked with drinks—Ben said he'd been shadowed by a black man, about six feet tall and 160 pounds, in a blue sweatsuit. The man didn't appear to be an athlete, and had no visible identification—there was nothing, in short, to indicate why he was allowed in the room. Ben had never seen him before, but the man never left his side, and was frequently in close and unsupervised proximity to the beers and juice Ben needed to drink to produce a urine sample. Ben added, however, that he hadn't seen the stranger do anything which might have led to his positive. (Beckett subsequently went to the lab to interview the officials on duty that Saturday. He said he was unable to find anyone to attest to the mystery man's presence.) Then, after 15 minutes of questioning, Ben left us and returned to his hotel.

During a break in our meeting before the "B" sample was opened, Beckett agreed that it was theoretically possible that Ben's sample might have been tainted even after the race, by someone tampering with Ben's drinks in the doping control room. Once inside the body, Beckett said, stanozolol was an extremely fast-acting drug that began to break down within 45 minutes to one hour. A sliver of doubt had entered the IOC's case, but I feared it wasn't yet enough to invalidate Ben's test on technical grounds—the way other athletes had been saved over the years. And I remained skeptical of a post-race drink-spiking scenario; such sabotage seemed to me too risky and uncertain of success.

At noon we went to the Shilla Hotel to enlist the aid of Richard Pound, a prominent Montreal attorney and IOC vice-president. Given the delicacy of his position, he might reasonably have referred us to someone else. But Pound was the only person with both the credibility to pursue a defence and the legal knowledge to mount one. To start off, he explained that any sabotage was pertinent only if it occurred *after* the race. The key to our case, he added, was not to identify a single suspect (who might turn out to be harmless), but to establish that the breaches in security in the doping control room left reasonable doubt about the test result.

Pound showed great courage in taking on his own organization. He went directly to see Juan Antonio Samaranch, the IOC president, and asked him to look into the security violations, since the Medical Commission might not rule impartially on its own lapses. According to Pound, Samaranch said he couldn't do it.

Meanwhile, I discovered that the media had been on to the story since noon that day, dimming my hopes for a quiet resolution. Since there were as yet no test results for Ben's "B" sample, and therefore no official finding, someone must have leaked the "A" sample results—another security violation. Although the IOC officials all advised us that the analysis of the "B" sample was merely a formality, since it came from the same specimen as the "A" sample, the leak—confirmed by Samaranch to Pound—provided further evidence of irregularities.

Our appeal meeting was scheduled for 10:00 P.M., by which time Park had confirmed that Ben's "B" sample contained stanozolol, as expected. While Pound and Stanish argued our case before about 20 members of the IOC Medical Commission, I waited in Pound's hotel suite with Carol Anne Letheren and the rest of the Canadian Olympic Association contingent. The mood was tense, some lame attempts at humour notwithstanding. At one point Carol Anne received an irate phone call from Lyle Makovsky, the top bureaucrat at the Canadian Ministry of Fitness and Amateur Sport, who was stuck in the lobby, since he lacked COA credentials. Makovsky demanded to know why he hadn't been informed of the test result earlier. Carol Anne coolly told him that he hadn't needed to know and that his presence could only bring more unwanted publicity. Noting that the hotel phones were tapped, she cut off further discussion. "I'm going to stand here until you come down and get me," Makovsky fumed. "Fine—stand there," Carol Anne replied.

As the hours passed, I became more optimistic; the commission must be split. Moreover, I knew that the IOC would be loathe to lose Ben and his record, and to set off the media inquisition that would surely follow. It was close to 1:00 A.M. Tuesday when Pound phoned the room with the bad news: Our appeal had been rejected, and Ben's positive was official. The commission would recommend that Ben be disqualified, a decision which the IOC's executive committee would be certain to uphold later that day.

Numbed by 20 hours of anxiety, I met Pound and the COA officials to commiserate at the hotel bar. We were joined by John Holt, general secretary to the International Amateur Athletic Federation, the world governing body for track and field and the IOC's most powerful constituent group. (Outside of the Olympics, which are run by the IOC, the IAAF sets rules and policies for international competition in track and field.) Dick Pound had done an outstanding job, Holt said, and his defence would surely have prevailed against the stanozolol positive. But in an unprecedented step initiated by Manfred Donike, the commission had also considered Ben's "endocrine profile," a measure of natural hormone levels which ostensibly showed that Ben had been using steroids for some time prior to the Olympics, making the question of sabotage moot. (According to IOC lab theory, natural hormone production would be depressed by long-term steroid use.)

I was dumbstruck; it was the first I'd ever heard of these profiles. They had never before been employed to confirm an athlete's drug use, nor would they be applied to any other doping case at Seoul. If such an analysis were reliable, why wasn't it used for everyone? And if it were too untried to be failsafe, how could it be used against Ben alone?

Only an endocrinologist could have countered the commission's eleventh-hour tactic. But Pound had no way of knowing he would need such an expert, since the commission failed to disclose its purported evidence in advance. The endocrine profile was a card they'd kept in their pocket until they were about to lose the hand.

Ben's reign as Olympic champion was over almost before it had begun; the fastest performance in the history of the world was now null and void. Ben would be stripped of his new world record. (His previous record, the 9.83 he'd set in Rome in 1987, would be allowed to stand—temporarily.) The IAAF would also suspend him from competition for two years, the prescribed penalty for first-time steroid offenders.

Despite the lateness of the hour, Canadian Olympic officials needed to reach Ben at his hotel and retrieve his medal before the news became public that morning. I drove through the pre-dawn chill to the Seoul Hilton with Carol Anne and Bill Stanish, and asked for a half-hour alone with Ben. Inside his hotel room, as I relayed the commission's decision, Ben's mother, Gloria, and his sister Jean were sobbing. "Oh my God, oh my God," Gloria Johnson kept repeating. Jamie Astaphan, the doctor who had supervised our sprint team's drug protocols for the past three years, was barely able to speak. I asked him if he knew of any way Ben might have taken stanozolol, or whether furazabol's metabolites might be confused with those of the more common steroid. Astaphan rejected either possibility.

Larry Heidebrecht, Ben's Virginia-based agent, looked ashen. He knew better than anyone just how much had been lost. All of Ben's major endorsement deals would be cancelled with the announcement of a positive test. (Heidebrecht later estimated that Ben's total loss would approach $10 million for 1989 alone, and $25 million over his career.)

Ben was the calmest person in the room. At 26, he'd been tempered by years of the most demanding competition and publicity. His emotional reserve—a quality that had made him such a great sprinter—now helped him keep his family from panicking. He hugged his mother and said, "Come on, Mom, nobody's died."

Carol Anne entered the suite with Dr. Stanish and asked for the gold medal. She'd grown fond of Ben since travelling with him for a Board of Trade meeting that March, and now she was weeping. With a blank expression, Ben handed over the gold-plated disk with its tricolour ribbon. He'd given the medal to his mother, and now it would pass to arch-rival Carl Lewis—the man Ben had beaten by four feet on the track.

After the officials left, Larry and I tried to plan our next move. We both felt that Ben should get out of Korea as soon as he could. I wanted him to lie low in Singapore or Jamaica until we could devise a course of action, but Ben would have none of it. "I'm not going to be pushed out of my house," he insisted. "I live in Canada and I'm going home." A flight to Toronto through New York was booked for that morning. Accompanied by a 50-strong security detail, Ben and his family were whisked through a chaotic scene at Kimpo Airport to board their plane, where they would be shrouded behind a curtain. Upon landing in Toronto, the Johnsons would remain huddled in the cockpit until the plane was empty, in a futile effort to avoid the clamouring reporters. Cheered at his stopover by his supporters in New York, Ben would be booed in his hometown.

At 10:00 A.M. Tuesday, with Ben already gone, the IOC's Michèle Verdier solemnly read a dry statement to a packed auditorium at the Olympic press centre: "The urine sample of Ben Johnson, Canada, athletics, 100 metres, collected on Saturday, 24th September 1988, was found to contain the metabolites of a banned substance, namely stanozolol, an anabolic steroid."

The media firestorm broke with full force, and the fallout was immediate. The Canadian politicians who'd been so quick to claim credit for Ben's achievements were even quicker to distance themselves. Within minutes of the IOC's announcement, Jean Charest, minister for fitness and amateur sport, citing "a national embarrassment," declared that Ben would never again run for Canada. (After widespread criticism that he had denied Ben due process, Charest later put any official action on hold until after a government inquiry.)

After being up all night, I felt drained and despondent. The COA had advised me to steer clear of its press conference later that morning and to leave the country as soon as possible. My instant notoriety could only hurt my seven remaining athletes in Seoul.

I left before noon on a Canadian Airlines flight which required a change of planes and a two-hour holdover in Vancouver. Shortly after I collapsed in my seat, the flight crew sent back a wonderful note to convey to Ben. They declared that he'd been unfairly singled out, that they stood behind him, and that they knew full well what was required to succeed in international sport.

In Vancouver, airline officials pulled me into a private waiting room. They'd found a seat for me on a different flight to Toronto, enabling me to dodge the horde of reporters who'd unearthed my original itinerary.

In Toronto I was escorted out of the customs area to a stairwell where my fiancée, Angé Coon, was waiting. We were ushered to a parking garage and drove away unseen.

In the wake of Ben's tragedy and my own hasty departure, most of my other athletes performed poorly in Seoul—whether out of emotional disarray, or concern that they might test positive as well. Mark McKoy, who should have won a silver or bronze in the 110-metre hurdles, finished seventh. He left Seoul before the 4x100-metre relay (in which each of four sprinters goes 100 metres), saying he was too depressed to compete. With alternates in Ben's and Mark's places, the relay team—a credible contender for the gold at full strength—finished out of the medals. Tracy Smith fouled out in the long jump. And in the women's 4x400-metre relay, an event in which Canada had taken the silver in Los Angeles four years before, the squad was eliminated by a dropped stick.

The shock waves of Ben's disqualification appeared to hit other athletes hard as well. An unusual number of medal contenders either failed to appear for their events or were eliminated early in their competitions—in many cases, no doubt, out of fear that they might meet Ben's fate.

The Whole Truth

Few public figures ever enjoyed such overwhelming adulation as did Ben in the immediate aftermath of his gold medal run. Fewer still were ever reviled with the bitterness that followed his disqualification. Ben carried the fast man's burden—the collective fantasy of all who watch and wonder what it must feel like to fly over the ground. If he stumbled under the load, *he* had failed *us*. And there was no question that Ben had stumbled in Seoul; in this context, it was almost irrelevant whether he'd been pushed.

The reaction was predictably strong in Canada, where Ben had become *the* sports hero in the wake of hockey god Wayne Gretzky's departure for Los Angeles, the redeeming highlight of a disappointing Olympic team effort. Shortly after Ben's disgrace became official, Prime Minister Brian Mulroney called it "a personal tragedy for Ben and his family and equally a moment of great disappointment for all Canadians." From breakfast tables to barrooms, throughout the country, the scandal was the leading topic of conversation. Canada had not won an Olympic gold medal on the track since Percy Williams captured the 100 metres in 1928. Now, after a few moments of glory, the nation's point of pride had been snatched away. The result was a muddle of public sentiments: shock, bewilderment, sympathy, and anger.

It was the latter emotion, unfortunately, that coloured the work of most of our newspaper pundits. *Their* sentiments ranged from the aggrieved ("How could Ben do this to us?") to the venomous, as in an *Ottawa Citizen* column headlined, "Thanks a Lot, You Bastard."

But the public stoning of Ben Johnson was scarcely less intense in other countries. Munich's *Abendzeitung* judged Ben "a doping sinner," while London's *Daily Mirror* headlined its story with a single accusing word: "Cheat!" In the United States, Anita DeFrantz, a member of the IOC, called Ben "a coward [who] used a crutch. To use drugs is cowardly, it's cheating, it's disgusting, it's vile." And in the analysis of *Newsday'*s John Jeansonne, Ben, Astaphan, and I were "dirty rotten scoundrels [who] botched the job and were caught, that's all."

This was old-fashioned journalism in the tabloid tradition. The biggest story in Olympic history required the worst knave (Ben), the most Faganesque coach (me), and the most malevolent witch doctor (Astaphan).

Though I understood how the press worked, I was amazed at how smoothly most of the world's track and field writers could suspend reality—how they could pretend that Ben's use of steroids was in any way unusual in elite sport. I'd known many of these journalists for years, and they were anything but naive. Like the national track federations, writers routinely protected their own countries' athletes from scandal. (At Rome in 1987, I had lunch with a prominent Italian sportswriter just after a sports physician had blown the whistle on several well-known athletes in a magazine exposé—a scoop ignored by every newspaper in the country. "What an idiot!" the sportswriter said of the doctor. "The day I write about drug use by Italians is the day the rest of the world cleans up, and not before.") It was only after Ben's news value diminished that the press felt compelled to look further afield. The results were most revealing:

* While Ben was easily the most celebrated athlete to fail a drug test in Seoul, he was not the only one. Ten other athletes from seven other nations tested positive for banned substances. The unfortunates ranged from Bulgarian weightlifters to an Afghan wrestler to a Polish hockey player—all the usual suspects. Ben's case was remarkable precisely *because* he was a first-magnitude star, the only one ever to be caught. It might be noted that Ben was also the only major player in Seoul who lacked the clout of a powerful national federation behind him, something taken for granted by top athletes from the United States, the Soviet Union, East and West Germany, Britain, and Italy. In November 1988, Dr. Tony Millar told an Australian Senate inquiry (a probe which heard evidence that up to 70 percent of Australia's international competitors had used drugs) that this handful of track powers strives to apply anti-doping sanctions most rigorously against those who can fight them least. "The people who don't matter are eliminated," testified Dr. Millar, formerly the chief medical officer for the Commonwealth Games Association. "Yes, if Ben Johnson had come from the U.S.S.R., he would have received a negative instead of positive dope test in Seoul."

*Park Jong Sei, the Seoul lab director, told *The New York Times* that as many as 20 other Olympic athletes tested positive but were cleared by votes of the IOC Medical Commission. Several of the votes were split—which might suggest that power politics, rather than objective scientific evidence, determines whether an athlete is ruined or reprieved. According to Dr. Millar's testimony, international officials "get together and discuss this matter—I'll vote for you if you vote for me."

* At the Dubin Inquiry, the commission empowered by Canada's federal government, West German sportscaster Bernd Heller testified to a conversation with Manfred Donike, one of the medical commissioners in charge of the Olympic lab. According to Heller, Donike revealed that *up to 80 percent* of male track and field athletes at Seoul had endocrine profiles reflecting previous steroid use. While Donike disputed the percentage figure on the stand, he acknowledged that an undisclosed proportion of the profiles were

indeed positive. No action was taken against any of these athletes, aside from Ben—an indication that the endocrine profile had yet to be accepted as a reliable test.

* Dr. Robert Voy, chief medical officer for the United States Olympic Committee in 1988, conceded in *The New York Times* that a majority of Olympic athletes used steroids in training. Even IAAF General Secretary John Holt, while insisting to the BBC that steroid use had been "blown up out of all proportion," went on to estimate that "between 30 and 40 percent of the athletes who are in the leading 20 in every event...take drugs."

Most of these revelations became public information within a year of the Seoul Olympics. Taken together, they demonstrated that Ben's case was special only because he got caught. Even today, however, most reporting on the incident continues to rest on the canard established in those first banner headlines of September 1988: that Ben was an exception and that his rivals—by implication, if not absolution—were clean. It is a pat morality play, and pure mythology, but it has stuck.

No News Is Good News

When we discovered that reporters had staked out my apartment, Angé and I found haven at a nearby Toronto hotel and checked in under her name. I was absolutely incognito—a tremendous frustration for the media. Canada's greatest international triumph had turned into its most grievous disappointment, and every news outlet in the country wanted to get to the man who had supposedly engineered it—"the missing link in the drug caper that has ruined many lives," according to *The Toronto Star*.

There was one bright spot: Canadian decathlete Dave Steen had won a bronze medal. A member of the University of Toronto track club, Steen had fallen out with his coach, Andy Higgins, in the fall of 1985, and had come to me to improve his speed and power, key factors in nine of his ten events. I had worked with Steen three times a week for the last three years, and now it had paid off. His success could go a long way toward re-establishing my credentials as a coach.

We remained at the hotel for two weeks and ventured out at our peril. When Angé dropped by the apartment to pick up some clothes, two reporters tailed her car on the way out, and she took them on a grand chase before losing them. The building's caretaker was under constant pressure. One television crew demanded that he unlock my apartment door for them, and he had to enlist one of my larger neighbours to throw them out. Another reporter actually began scaling the balconies at the back of the building to reach my ninth-floor apartment. On two occasions, Angé arrived to find my apartment door inexplicably unlocked. Finally she boiled over. "Why don't you leave the guy alone?" she told the stake-out contingent. "His mother has cancer." With that, an especially enterprising journalist began phoning the local cancer wards until he reached my mother's room and began harassing her for information. She was upset; I was appalled.

To get away from our pursuers, we took a trip to Angé's parents' home in Belle River, a small town near Windsor, Ontario, only to find just how far the long arm of the press could reach. *The New York Times* had already searched out my future in-laws in its quest for background information. At Paddy's, a local gas station which also served coffee at a four-stool counter, the *Times* reporter had brandished pictures of myself and Ben, asking if anyone had spotted us in the vicinity.

On the highway between Belle River and Toronto, we stopped at a McDonald's, and the woman at the counter asked for my autograph. When I told my mother about it, she laughed and warned me not to get too excited. "They used to ask for John Dillinger's autograph, too," she said.

On September 30, in a column in *The Toronto Sun*, I read that Dave Steen had startled Andy Higgins by embracing him after the decathlon medal ceremony and saying, "I owe you a lot, coach." Now it was clear: Steen would bury our association and credit the coach he'd left three years before.

After a few days I began to regroup and think about the future. I held no illusions of returning to the sport. My hope was to expose the sabotage in Seoul, if that's what it had been, and to move on from there.

Early on, I received an offer from an international publishing group. In return for exclusive rights to our inside story, they would pay a package of $1.6 million (U.S.) to me, Jamie Astaphan, and Angella Issajenko. But we decided to turn the offer down. On October 5th, the federal government established its commission of inquiry into the use of drugs and banned practices in Canadian sport, to be headed by Charles Dubin, Ontario's associate chief justice. I decided that I would wait to speak until I was called as a witness.

I knew that I needed a high-powered trial lawyer; I retained Roy McMurtry, former Ontario attorney general and high commissioner to London. Our hope was for Ben to be represented by Bob Armstrong, who'd worked extensively on other commissions of inquiry, and to co-ordinate our legal strategies. (Armstrong was later selected as chief counsel for the Commission.) At this point, however, we were unable to get through to Ben, as his phone had been disconnected; we learned after the fact that he had hired Ed Futerman, a local attorney. But Ben's line of defence had already begun to emerge through public statements by such IOC heavyweights as Juan Antonio Samaranch and Dick Pound—the people who would ultimately decide his athletic fate. "Johnson probably wouldn't know what a steroid is," Pound had told the press. "His body may be guilty, but his mind is innocent." The doyens of the sport continued to hope that Ben could somehow be exonerated—not merely to salve his nation's wounds ("Say It Ain't So, Ben," one headline pleaded), but to restore track and field's pre-eminent star attraction. If supporting characters like Astaphan and me could be painted as having coerced an innocent athlete into taking drugs, Ben might yet be saved.

Just one week after Seoul, Ben took the bait. After rejecting a $500,000 (U.S.) offer from the German weekly *Stern* to tell his story there first, he put out a statement that was published October 1st in *The Toronto Sun*. "I have never knowingly taken illegal drugs nor have had illegal drugs administered to me," Ben declared. At a press conference three days later, he repeated that he had "never, ever, knowingly taken illegal drugs." While I empathized with Ben and the impossible position he'd been placed in, I was shaken and hurt by this falsehood. If Ben stuck to these statements, they would support the theory that I had deceived him by giving him steroids without his knowledge or assent—a scenario that would lead to criminal charges against me.

Angella Issajenko perceived Ben's statement as a betrayal, and she was furious with her old teammate. On October 9th, she took him on in an explosive interview with *The Toronto Star*. "Ben takes steroids, I take steroids," Angella told the reporter. "Jamie [Astaphan] gives them to us, and Charlie isn't a scientist, but he knows what's happening." Everyone involved, she made clear, understood exactly what was going on. "When you play games, you live by codes," she told *The Toronto Sun*. "If you make a mistake or something goes wrong, you accept the consequences. You don't back down and slaughter the people you were in league with from the beginning."

For the time being, I restricted myself to a brief public statement, as approved by my attorney. I neither admitted nor denied that Ben had taken steroids, but suggested that foul play was involved. Ben's positive, I said, "can only be explained by a deliberate manipulation of the testing process." Dr. Astaphan, by contrast, had opted for a total stonewall; in a September 28th interview on CBC television, he maintained that he'd never given steroids or any other banned drugs to Ben.

Meanwhile, Ben was a virtual hostage in his suburban Toronto home, and he was beginning to fray. During the second week after his return, a motorist complained that Ben had pointed a gun at him when caught in traffic; a police search turned up a starter's pistol—the "gun" in question—in Ben's black Porsche. Ben pleaded guilty to common assault, and received a conditional discharge and 12 months' probation.

A few weeks later I was rocked by news of another sort. The Dubin Inquiry had submitted for laboratory analysis a sample of the injectable steroid, provided by Angella, that members of my sprint group had been using for the past three years. In November, the lab issued its report—and revealed that the sample was *not* furazabol (the untestable steroid we had known as Estragol). It was, rather, *stanozolol*, the same commonly used steroid that had surfaced in Ben's drug test at Seoul. My confusion—and dismay—was compounded. I would never have allowed my sprinters to use an injectable known to the IOC—I would have feared the possibility that its metabolites wouldn't clear their systems in time. (Oral steroids, which we had relied on before Astaphan introduced us to "Estragol" in 1985, clear the body much faster than injectables.)

This revelation failed to solve the mystery of Ben's positive, however. As far as I knew, he had received his last injection on August 28th in Toronto, or 26 days before the 100-metre final. There should have been ample time for the drug to clear, based on our past experience. Using the same steroid, Ben had tested clean on 29 previous occasions, often with clearance times of less than 26 days. In several instances, he'd taken an injection as close as 13 or 14 days before a meet. Why had he tested positive this time?

Amid this swirl of conflicting stories, I bided my time, and waited for the Dubin Inquiry, which was expected to convene early the following year. I would try to demonstrate that Ben had won on a level playing field in Seoul, and that his spectacular accomplishment should be returned to the record books. Over the next six months, I would prepare obsessively for my eight days in the Inquiry's witness box, retracing every step I'd taken as a runner and coach over 25 years. I would summon up a career rich in friends and adversaries, in breakthroughs and setbacks.

In the process, I would seek to rebuild my reputation as the coach who had forged one of the world's leading sprint teams, whose runners had set 32 world records and won 9 Olympic medals, and who had, by the unwritten rules of my day, developed the fastest man in history.

For years I had been a good soldier. I had kept the conspiracy of silence that governs international track, a see-no-evil world where high-minded condemnations of drug use coexist with the cynical protection of doped-up superstars. But silence wouldn't work any more—not for me and not for Ben. It was finally time to speak up.

The Schoolboy

I always loved to run. For a boy growing up in the 1950s, in Rosedale, an affluent Toronto neighbourhood, the activity held one great attraction: I was good at it. In other areas, my gifts were not so clear. In team sports I was a total bust. I had no hand-eye co-ordination to speak of, and in schoolyard games I would be picked next to last, just before the fat kid.

Although running came naturally to me, my first formal sprint was inauspicious. In a charge of 30 weaving first-graders in a district competition, I was cut off by two kids and trapped behind the crowd. (My classmate Jack Robbins was leading until he dropped his handkerchief, and ceded the race when he stopped to pick it up.) But from second grade on I won the district championship every year.

I was lucky to have parents who supported my athletic pursuits. My father was a former ice dancer who developed the "Canasta Tango," which remains a compulsory routine in international competition to this day. He was also an artist who worked in the figurative tradition, despite the commercial trend towards abstracts. He was stubborn in pursuing his passions—a trait he passed on to me. My mother was a Maryland-born teacher, the daughter of the history chairman at the U.S. Naval Academy at Annapolis. From her I inherited a love of reading and the high-strung temperament that is part of every sprinter's makeup.

In high school I won every 100-yard dash I entered. For summer competition I joined the Don Mills Track Club in Toronto in 1964, when I was 15, and, though the coaches there knew little about the finer points of sprinting, I continued to improve. I won five national age-class championships and set a Canadian juvenile (under 18) record of 9.6 seconds in the 100 yards. Though I'd also won titles in the 220, the 100 was always my favourite event—the blue-ribbon competition, the one which told who was fastest.

The 100-metre champion rules the most elemental of contests, the truest test for sheer speed. In the very first Olympics, held in ancient Greece in 776 B.C., the single competition was a sprint. The event is seemingly (if deceptively) simple and literally straightforward. It crosses cultural lines like no other, and is by far the most competitive—and the most glamorous—Olympic endeavour. More than 160 nations contested the 100 in 1988, as compared to about 80 in swimming and 30 in gymnastics. From Europe to South America and almost everywhere in between, hundreds of millions of children line up in schoolyards and *run*, to see who will finish first. The losers switch to other sports or become milers or marathoners, milieus where gamesmanship and grinding effort can compensate for more limited physical gifts. The winners race on, in ever narrowing fields. They start in local clubs, then move on to provincial and national meets. A few might make their national teams and enter international competition, ranging from two-country dual meets to the Olympics. Fewer still might be invited to participate in the IAAF/Mobil Grand Prix meets in Europe, the most competitive and prestigious track circuit in the world. Only the very best will make it to the Olympic final of the 100 metres, and then one man will stand alone. The world's fastest human belongs to everyone—and when I was 15 years old, no other title seemed quite so royal.

Running became my obsession. I followed the career of the American Bob Hayes—the fastest human of that day, and the Olympic gold medallist in 1964—the way other teenagers followed

Bobby Hull or Willie Mays. My great thrill came in 1966, at the Canadian national championships in Edmonton, where I met one of my boyhood heroes: Harry Jerome, the fastest man in Canada.

Jerome was a freak of nature, an aberration. You could say he was the greatest sprinter Canada had yet produced, except that Canada had nothing to do with it. He competed years before Sport Canada was established, at a time when his country provided its athletes with neither financial help nor technical support. The son of a Saskatchewan railway porter, Jerome showed just how far a fast man could go it alone.

Jerome was unknown outside Canada when he tied the world record at 10-flat for the 100 metres in 1960, as a freshman at the University of Oregon. He was an inexperienced kid, not nearly ready to face the best veteran sprinters in the world. But the press anointed him as the nation's great hope to win a gold medal at the 1960 Olympics in Rome. He was sent there in September, after a summer in Canada without coaching or high-level competition. But Jerome was good, and too young to know his limits. He was leading his semi-final when his lack of preparation betrayed him; he pulled a hamstring and limped to a stop.

Jerome discovered that a star disappoints the Canadian public at his peril. Long after Rome, he was dogged by the press as a "choke." But he overcame this abuse to notch three more world records over the next two years, and in 1962 was ranked first in the world for 220 yards by *Track & Field News*. He also became one of only two men ever to beat the brilliant Hayes in the 100. In the fall of 1962, after another wasted summer in Canada, Jerome travelled to the Commonwealth Games at Perth, Australia. He was moving full-bore in the 100 yards when his spikes ripped away from his shoe. He hyperextended his leg and ruptured his quadriceps, the set of long muscles at the front of the thigh; a tendon was torn from the knee joint. Jerome landed in surgery and was still in the hospital when he came across a Vancouver newspaper. He was reduced to tears by a banner headline: "Jerome Quits Again."

The Games at Perth should have marked the end of his career— his injured thigh would always be more than an inch smaller around than his other one—but Jerome fought back once more. Though he would never run as powerfully again, he improved his start and worked his way back to the top: the bronze medal in the 100 metres in the 1964 Olympics; the gold in the Commonwealth Games of 1966 and the Pan Ams of 1967; yet another world record for the 100 yards. He remained world-ranked from 1960 through 1968, a rare feat of longevity.

For all of his accomplishments, however, Jerome remained a voice in the wilderness. By advocating public financing for athletes, he alienated a sports establishment content to emulate Britain's upper-class amateur tradition. By the time the country came to accept his ideas, Jerome was a sick man; he died of a brain lesion at the age of 42.

Stanford

As I approached the end of high school, I knew my destiny pointed
south, to the United States. The Canadian universities had little
in the way of indoor training facilities and virtually no track
scholarships. America represented adventure and opportunity, and
I wanted to be part of it.

When Stanford began recruiting me, it all sounded promising:
the California climate, the best competition, and not least the
school's head coach, Payton Jordan, who had developed Larry
Questad into the 1963 National Collegiate Athletic Association
100-yard champion. Jordan secured his reputation in 1965, when
his 440-yard relay team set a world record and Stanford placed
a surprising second in the NCAA track and field championships.
He'd already been named head coach for the 1968 U.S. Olympic
track team. I had my own Olympic dreams, and I hoped he would
help me realize them. He would be my mentor, I thought, my first
real coach. I left home for Stanford in the fall of 1967.

Jordan had starred as a sprinter at the University of Southern
California in the 1940s, and he still cut an impressive figure:
ruggedly handsome, ramrod straight, and terrifically fit for a man
in his 50s. There was no question that he knew his stuff. But

it seemed to me that his heart was no longer in it; I found him inconsistent in his attentions and follow-up. In the wake of his mid-sixties breakthroughs, he'd turned down the head coach's job at the University of Southern California, only to see his good work at Stanford rewarded by a crippling series of budget cuts. By the time I'd arrived, he was left with only three scholarships a year. Jordan knew his team would never reprise its Cinderella story of 1965, and thought longingly of USC's advantages, including an unlimited number of scholarships and an admissions department which could be flexible where athletes were concerned.

Training time at Stanford was an organized riot. Many athletes devised their own work-outs as they went along. The lazy ones did so little that they lacked the most basic conditioning. Others, like myself, ran themselves into the ground. Overstressed and underprepared, I had one muscle strain after another through my sophomore and junior years.

In fairness, the chaos in collegiate track was not unique to Stanford. The great majority of college coaches failed to produce a single high-performance athlete. A handful of high-powered NCAA programs—at UCLA, USC, Tennessee, and a few other universities—turned out all the best performers, year after year. But even the top programs weren't all that well organized; at USC, I knew runners on the same team who trained at different tracks. In contrast to the situation in Europe, where the various national federations structured meticulous training plans to allow their athletes to peak at the most important meets, American collegians skimped on practice and relied instead on the most rigorous competitive schedule in the world. They could simply run themselves into form at their competitions—but only if they didn't kill themselves training in between. Beginning in February, they'd have two or three races every weekend, and by June they'd be flying. In such a haphazard system, however, only a few would thrive. The super talents sailed through, since they could win going easy or going hard. For the rest of us, our development was a matter of chance.

One exception to this rule of anarchy was Bud Winters' program at San Jose State. A relaxation therapist who'd trained Navy fliers during the Second World War, Winters was both a fine technician and a great innovator—an early advocate of low-volume speed training and a pioneer in designing individualized training programs for his athletes. While a few of his athletes—notably John Carlos, Tommie Smith, and Lee Evans—went on to become stars, Winters' sprint team also had incredible depth; at one point he had seven runners going 9.4 or better in the 100 yards. The world had never seen such a stable of sprinters, nor would it again.

It was in my junior year at Stanford that I first dabbled with the notion of performance-enhancing drugs. One weekend I was slotted to run the dreaded 440 yards, invariably an ordeal for me. I'd heard that amphetamines could delay the onset of fatigue, and decided to give them a try. The drugs weren't exactly scarce at Stanford, where every dorm light would be blazing at 5:00 A.M. during exam week. An hour before the race, I popped a five-milligram Dexedrine tablet. By the time I'd gone 250 yards, I knew the stuff wasn't working, and I finished as miserably as usual. I tried Dexedrine one more time that year, in a 220-yard race toward the end of the regular season, and ran poorly once again. It was my last experiment with speed, though I didn't blame the drug. If you're not prepared by your training, I concluded, *nothing* will help you.

I later learned that a number of elite athletes used amphetamines to great effect. In 1976, Mike Mercer, a Canadian shot-putter who'd attended college in Utah, related a story about a U.S. meet in which he had competed years before. Shortly before the competition, Mercer had run into a long-jumper who seemed depressed. The jumper had reached close to 25 feet in high school, but hadn't improved in the four years since then. Feeling compassionate, Mercer told me, he handed over a 25-milligram Dexedrine/Benzedrine tablet—five times stronger than my dose—and instructed the jumper to take it 45 minutes before his event. The next day, as Mercer waited in the shot-putters' area for his turn, the victorious jumper came running through the middle of the competition, shouting, "Mike, Mike! Twenty-six feet!"

My 1970 collegiate season had no such happy ending; it was a disaster from start to finish. That summer I resolved to do something drastic. I called Percy Duncan.

The Mentor

I had called Percy once before, on a friend's reference, a week before the 1968 Olympic trials in Toronto. He advised me on how to relax and supplied a good "taper schedule"—a series of work-outs of diminishing volume—for that last week. In the trials I ran a wind-aided 10.4 and finished an unexpected second to Harry Jerome. The experiment was a success, but I was still reluctant to swallow Percy's philosophies whole. Everything he said was so different from all I had heard before. Percy was asking me to shelve all my preconceptions about running, and I wasn't ready. I feared losing what I already had.

But by June of 1970, I had nothing more to lose. My new mentor was a tall, well-muscled man in his mid-50s who looked 20 years younger. A native of Guyana, Percy had tied the world record for 100 yards in the 1940s, and hadn't lost his athlete's conditioning. He was working in the complaints department of a Toronto department store, but sprinting remained his first love.

Percy was a superb teacher, perpetually jovial and endlessly patient—a good deal more patient than I was. When we finally got together, at a municipal stadium in Toronto, I had only seven weeks to prepare for the Eastern Canadian Championships in late

July, the first summer meet of importance. After I told Percy about my previous hamstring problem, he said, "Come on, let me look at your muscles." For Percy, a "look" meant a full-hour massage, and this in itself was something new for me. When track coaches deny the value of massage, I suspect an ulterior motive. If they acknowledged its benefits, they might actually have to *do* it—and massage is hard, grunting work. In three years at Stanford I'd never been massaged by Payton Jordan or anyone else. Now I found what I'd been missing. Aside from its regenerative qualities, massage is the best possible diagnostic tool, the only way to gauge a runner's muscle tone, which in turn defines his state of readiness—or his vulnerability to injury.

When Percy was finished that first day, he didn't like what he'd found. "Go home," he told me.

"What do you mean?" I said.

"Your muscles aren't ready to train, they're all tight and knotted," he replied. "Come back tomorrow."

We repeated that scene for four straight days, until I could barely contain my frustration. But Percy was adamant: I would run when I was ready, and no sooner. On the fifth day he was finally satisfied. "All right," he said, "now you're going to learn how to walk." That entire work-out consisted of walking and light jogging, with Percy watching my rhythm and making sure I stayed relaxed.

On the sixth day my teacher deemed me ready: "Let's have a look at you." To gauge my maximum speed, he set up two markers 20 metres apart on the track, then put me through "finishing drills." I would hit top speed when I reached the first marker and maintain velocity until I passed the second one, then ease up. (You can't maintain maximum speed for much more than 20 metres, anyway.) When I was through, Percy concluded that my top speed was good, but my overall race was weak. This conformed to my own experience; I usually felt strong at the beginning and end of the 100 metres, but in the middle I'd often sag.

Then the real work began. Much of it was aimed at improving my mechanics. Instead of addressing my overall technique, Percy focused on a very few key components, and only one of them at a time. If I performed these correctly, he believed, everything else would fall into place. He set me in front of a mirror to practise a proper arm swing: hands pumping up to eye level, arms bent at the elbows at 90-degree angles. To keep my hips loose and mobile (a problem for most sprinters), he had me run along a lane-divider line. If I was relaxed and my hips were moving properly, my stride would naturally swing slightly toward the centre, with one foot landing in front of the other on the line. Each of these drills made sense to me, and I could feel the results when I ran.

Percy taught me the difference between running and sprinting—that while you run *on* the ground, you sprint *over* it, with the briefest possible foot contact. It's like the spinning of a bicycle wheel; a sharp slap of the hand will impart more speed to the wheel than would a more prolonged stroke. The strongest sprinters spend the least time in pushing along the ground. They focus instead on moving their legs up and down, and are barely conscious of how their force is translated into horizontal impetus. They feel ease rather than power in their motion, since they overcome resistive forces—ground and air, gravity and inertia—with so little difficulty.

I had long assumed that more work was better and had always trained until I could train no longer. Percy was the first coach I'd encountered who understood that *less* was more: that too much work saps an athlete, and that you keep a runner sharpest (and most likely to excel in competition) with *low* volumes of practice. At Stanford I would run all-out for up to 320 metres at a stretch, but Percy's maximum speed drills never exceeded 70 metres. More typically, I'd go 20 metres fast out of the blocks, then easy for 60 metres, then hard again for 20 metres, in sets of six. Intensity was more important than volume. At the same time, Percy stressed the value of recovery between high-intensity sprints. An ordinary coach might tell you to walk back to the starting line after a sprint and go again, but Percy made me rest up to ten minutes between five- or ten-second speed drills.

Percy saw no point in running at intermediate speeds, which he thought would tighten your muscles without honing your power. He wanted his runners moving fast or slow—nothing in between.

That summer I ran as far as 300 metres only once each day, at the close of the work-out, and I ran it so slowly (about 42 seconds) that it functioned as a cool-down. Overall, I logged only 60 percent as much volume as I had at Stanford.

At first I was apprehensive. This *couldn't* be enough work. After one especially brief session, Percy told me I was through for the day. I insisted that I wasn't tired—that I could go on. "Yeah?" he said. "You come back tomorrow and tell me if you think you could have done any more." As soon as I got up the next morning, stiff and sore, I knew he was right; I realized how much work I had actually put in. The insidious thing about speed training is that you can't feel it until hours *after* your drills. The delayed reaction lands many sprinters in trouble, unless their coach watches them closely and knows when to call a halt.

Percy and I trained six days a week. As the meet date approached, I wondered whether we could afford the day off—why not work on Sunday as well? But Percy vetoed my proposal: "The Lord made the world in six days, and on the seventh He rested. Do you think you could do better than that?"

For all of Percy's advances, we made one major mistake during our summer together. Like virtually everyone else in North America, we were doing daily, maximum-velocity speed work—at much lower volumes than the norm, granted, but daily speed work nonetheless. We didn't know what Bud Winters and the top Europeans had discovered: that a sprinter needs 48 hours to recharge the central nervous system after going at top speed.

Even so, five weeks of training with Percy left me sounder and fresher than I'd ever been. At a minor meet I ran a 10.5 in the 100 metres despite a stiff headwind. I knew I was primed to do even better two weeks later, when I travelled to Halifax for the Eastern Canadian Championships. My first heat was so easy it seemed a joke, and I guessed I'd won it in 10.8. When the results were posted, I found out I'd run 10.4—a new personal best.

The finals confirmed Percy's brilliance: I won in a wind-aided 10.1 seconds. (The worldwide standard for an allowable tailwind is

2 metres per second, or about 4.5 miles per hour; any performance time achieved with a tailwind exceeding 2 metres is considered "wind-aided", and cannot count as a record, since reduced wind resistance makes for faster times.) I was far faster than ever before—I was in a new zone. I went on to win the 200 metres, a race where I'd feared for my endurance, given my limited-distance speed training. I was timed in 20.8 seconds, an astounding half-second better than my personal best going in.

The conditions weren't so favourable in the 1970 Canadian National Championships two weeks later (it was raining in Winnipeg, with a headwind), but the results were the same. I ran 10.4 and 21-flat in the two sprints, and won them both without trouble. The 100 metres also marked the first time I'd beaten Harry Jerome. My old boyhood hero was 30 years old, at the end of his great career.

Beating Jerome was bittersweet for me. I'd gotten to know the man earlier that summer, when he'd trained with me at Birchmount Stadium in suburban Toronto. I'd asked him every question I could think of, and he proved generous with his time and expertise.

Jerome couldn't explain how he got ready for a meet, since he trained intuitively, varying his work from day to day. He worked hard, but within his capacity. With his acute self-awareness, he usually quit before he overdid it. But technique was another matter—on this subject, Jerome was a teaching virtuoso. Aside from his experience as a world-class runner, he had researched the subject in rare depth. (He'd written his Ph.D. thesis on starting technique.) He made one central observation—that when a sprinter tries to accelerate, he must be patient above all. There are two variables to consider: the time warp within a sprinter's mind, where each second drags like ten; and the fact that it takes a moment for your body to transmit your acceleration onto the track. Before the heightened rhythm kicks in, there will be an agonizing pause. But a runner must keep faith. If he can stay under control, he'll do well, if only because his rivals are likely to lose *their* composure. But if he panics and pushes harder, he'll get tight and defeat himself.

Much of Jerome's advice overlapped with Percy's. Both stressed sound mechanics, and in particular the importance of the sprinter's arms. The conventional wisdom declared that sprinters should strive to lengthen their stride out of the blocks, but Harry and Percy denounced this as nonsense. If you concentrated on your arms and your hand position, they told me, your feet would automatically land in the right spots.

The summer of 1970 changed my life. I had been fantastically fortunate, for Harry and Percy were more than the best track minds in Canada—they were the *only* minds. In the years to come, their training would make me a better coach. I was able to help the likes of Ben Johnson and Angella Issajenko because I'd approached the world-class level myself. I knew what good sprinting felt like, as well as the toll that it took on your system. I could tell other athletes both how to move and when to stop. But I couldn't have known these things unless Harry and Percy had first shown me, because I never would have gotten fast enough. I'm not saying it's impossible to coach world-class sprinters without having done it yourself. But it's certainly much harder.

Olympic Dreams

In my senior year at Stanford I came into my own. I essentially coached myself, but stuck with Percy's summer lessons as best I could. I steered clear of serious injury for a change—no doubt because I wasn't training quite so hard. I swept most of my sprints, and at season's end I won the team award for compiling the most dual-meet points.

In June of 1971, at the age of 22, I ran a 10.1 in the 100 metres at the Pan Am trials in Vancouver, the fastest race of my life. I was training well going in, and felt supremely easy and fluid that day. My stride was open, my arms and legs fully extended, my knees up—everything came together, and I won by six yards. My effort placed me fifth on the world list of performances that year.

The Pan Am Games, held in Cali, Colombia, attracted the toughest 100-metre field I'd ever faced: from Jamaica, Don Quarrie, who would tie the world record for the 200 metres at this meet, and Lennox Miller, the 1968 Olympic silver medallist; from the U.S., Del Meriwether, who'd just run a wind-aided 9.0 to win the 100 yards at the American championships; from Cuba, Pablo Montes and Hermes Ramirez, who had teamed to help win the silver medal in the 4x100 relay at the 1968 Olympics. Judging from my performance in the trials, I felt I had a chance to medal, even at this level. Cali's 5,000-foot altitude is ideal for sprinting, and in practice I went very fast—too fast. After recording several personal bests at 70 metres, I suffered a slight hamstring strain four days before the race. Despite my injury, I finished fifth in the final, which was won by Quarrie. (I ran 10.31 there in my first experience with electronic timing, now the standard format for all major meets. The electronic timer begins instantly with the firing of the gun; a hand-held watch, by contrast, begins only after the person holding it reacts to the gun and pushes a finger down—on average, .24 seconds later. My performance in Cali, therefore, was as fast as my hand-timed personal best at the Pan Am trials.)

After the Pan Ams, my confidence was stronger than ever. But while I believed I could hold my own at the world level, I never dreamed that I could make a living at my game. (Like other North Americans, I didn't know that many of my European counterparts were being paid under the table for meet appearances.) I decided to return to the track, however, for one more year and one last challenge: the Olympics.

Back in Toronto that summer, I resumed my training with Percy, won the nationals for the second consecutive year, and beat the young Italian star, Pietro Mennea, at a dual meet in Sardinia. But reality struck when I returned home to prepare for the 1972 season. It was tough, as always, to stay in shape through the Canadian winter. I visited California in March of 1972 for three meets, then accepted invitations to compete in Barbados and Trinidad, and won in both places. (Invitational meets are a special blessing for athletes, since all expenses are paid.) I began rounding into form, but slid back again after returning to Toronto that May; CTFA officials had failed to arrange a single international competition during that pre-Olympic season. With Percy working overtime at his real job, it was hard for us to get together, and my training suffered. I ran several 10.2s in competition, but couldn't match my 10.1 of the year before.

The *coup de grâce* came at Canada's Olympic trials in Toronto in July 1972, a month before the Games. I'd strained my quadriceps the Thursday before the meet. It wasn't serious, and I'd have quickly recovered if I'd been allowed to skip the trials—a reasonable proposition, since I'd already met the Olympic standard of 10.3 more than a dozen times and hadn't lost to a Canadian since 1969. But there was no precedent for a bye, and I ran in three races within four hours. I limped home third in the final—but the Canadian Olympic Association nonetheless selected me (as was their prerogative) for the Olympic team, passing over the two who had beaten me. I was bound for Munich, ready or not.

Even before I arrived in Germany in late August, I had a dark feeling about these Games. Running at the Olympics had never been an end in itself for me; my dream was to be a *contender*. But from the time I arrived, it was obvious that I—along with my Canadian teammates and the rest of the athletic Third World—had been cast as extras. The International Olympic Committee needed us to swell the fields and force its stars into extra rounds of competition, a boon to ticket sales. I'd been competitive at the Pan Ams, but in Munich the ground had shifted: I just wasn't one of the players.

A few days before my event, Lionel Pugh, Canada's head coach, forced me to run in a preparatory meet. It was cold and gusty that night, with a driving rain. No major sprinters ran in such conditions, but I had no choice; Pugh was the boss, and he insisted. After a drenching one-hour warm-up and another hour's delay, I won my 200-metre section in a pedestrian 21.3 seconds. After the race, as I was wringing out my sweats, Pugh offered his critique: "Looks like you're out of shape." I didn't have the energy to strangle him.

In Munich the awesome quality—and financial backing—of the world's leading track programs was manifest. Here was the state of the art—in training, in preparation, in technical sophistication. I saw the Soviet Valery Borzov, the eventual double gold medallist, come to the track with an entourage of five people to arrange his blocks, to measure and time his every drill. I saw the Italian Pietro Mennea, the man I'd beaten in 1971, enter the Games in absolute peak form, looking nothing like the runner of the year before. These stars, and others like them, were totally ready, completely confident—the beneficiaries of organized efforts and time-tested programs.

Percy and Harry had lent me the technical ability to compete at this level, but I had no annual plan, no logically spaced sequence of competitions leading up to my ultimate test. Years later, as a coach, I would schedule five to seven tune-ups for a 100-metre runner before a major meet. But in 1972, I had no clue as to how to arrange for these competitions.

The facilities in Munich underlined the Europeans' edge. There were tracks of all surfaces—dirt, grass, and synthetic. The big national teams had weight rooms staffed around the clock with specialists and masseurs. Starters were available for practice at all times.

The 1972 Olympics revealed one more area where sophisticated training programs had a leg up on the rest of the world: the use of anabolic steroids. Prior to Munich, my futile flings with Dexedrine aside, I was a pharmaceutical illiterate. I knew that anabolics were around—particularly Dianabol, the athletes' steroid of choice at the time. I'd overheard throwers talking about how big they wanted to get—but at 185 pounds, I had no desire to get any bigger. I had no idea that steroids had other potential benefits for sprinters.

I was passing time in the Olympic Village when I ran into Gary Power, a non-competing American hurdler. He asked me if I were taking steroids and was surprised when I told him I wasn't. "Are you crazy?" he said. "Why not?" I told him I couldn't see how they could help me—and besides, couldn't they test for these things? Power explained that there were no tests for anabolic steroids (they would not be explicitly banned until 1975), and that they'd become essential for sprinting and hurdling events at this level. As I listened, I felt foolish in my ignorance, but also intrigued.

After lunch I was visiting Laurie D'Arcy, a New Zealand sprinter whom I'd met in Tokyo, and his roommate, the thrower Robin Tait, when a huge form ambled by and filled the doorway. It was Jay

Silvester, then the top American discus thrower, who would go on to win the silver medal.

"Hey, Robin," Silvester said, "you got any spare Dianabol? I'm out." Tait casually tossed him a small bottle. Silvester opened it, shook out a few tablets, popped them into his mouth, then stuck the bottle in his rear pocket. "Thanks, man," he said, and walked away.

I was impressed. If steroids worked as well as advertised, I knew I was going to try them before long. I gathered all the information available—which was plenty, since athletes had no fear of exposure, and since most rivals of importance were already users. During my two weeks in Munich, I heard story after story about names and cases—many of them big names, including Olympic champions. I learned that steroids were especially helpful for sprinters in major competitions, to surmount the physical stress of multiple rounds of heats—situations where I had always been weakest.

The picture was further clarified in Munich by the imposing figure of Renate Stecher, East Germany's top woman sprinter. I had never seen a woman like her in my life. She looked bigger than Borzov—and more muscular, too. As I watched her win the 100 and 200, both in world-record times—years before she was named as a steroid user by a member of the East German Olympic Committee—I saw proof of the impact of anabolics. (British authorities and athletes were similarly impressed, to the point where they demanded action from the IOC following these Olympics—a campaign that foreshadowed the steroid ban three years later.)

Unfortunately, my enlightenment came too late to help me on the track. By my race day, September 1st, I'd fallen prey to self-consciousness. I no longer hoped to make the final. I prayed only that I wouldn't embarrass myself. In past races, I had thrived on a rush of adrenaline just before my event; on this day, I felt numbed, strangely passive.

As I observed the heats preceding my own and followed the posted results, I felt even worse. A fast time is the loser's consolation, but it wasn't going to happen for me in Munich. The stadium track's synthetic coating hadn't cured properly, so they'd had to lay a new one just before the Games. The surface was softer and slower than anticipated, and I was shocked by the heat times—respectable runners were finishing in the 10.50s.

In my morning heat my quadriceps was sore, but I qualified in 10.65. At 4:00 P.M. I returned to the official call area, a room crowded with more than 40 other quarter-finalists, to glumly await my turn. The place was in an uproar. The two top-ranked American sprinters, Rey Robinson and Eddie Hart, had been misinformed by an official and arrived at the track after their quarters had run. Both had been legitimate medal contenders, and now they were disqualified—four years of work undone by another man's blunder. Hart, who'd been considered the top threat to Borzov, sat down on a bench with tears running down his cheeks. I knew Eddie from his days at Berkeley and felt genuinely sorry for him (though I might have been more ambivalent if he'd been slotted for *my* quarter-final). Meanwhile, the third American, Robert Taylor, reached the call area barely in time for his race, and rushed out to his blocks without a warm-up. But Taylor kept his poise. He deliberately false-started—allowing him to jog out to the wire and do a few stretches on the way back to the blocks. Then, as Valery Borzov tried to lure him into a speed duel (and a possible injury) by blasting a 10.07, a world sea-level record, Taylor responded with a swift 10.16 of his own—a remarkable effort under the circumstances. The American was loose enough to avoid pulling a muscle, and ultimately took the silver medal.

My own race offered no such drama. I could feel the quadriceps worsening with every stride, and finished last in 10.51. My time would have been good enough to advance me to the semis from two slower quarter-finals, but I couldn't have run again, anyway. My Olympics were over.

I told Paul Poce, the coach responsible for my event, that my injury would bar my running in the 200 metres. After my 200 heat went without me, I was called into a coaches' meeting—and onto the carpet.

"You are guilty of the worst crime an athlete can commit," intoned a solemn Lionel Pugh. "You failed to run in an event in which you were entered in the Olympic Games." I argued that I had fulfilled my obligation by informing Poce of my problem, but I couldn't make any headway. Team officials told the press that I had been "disciplined" for my alleged offence.

Munich was not a great Olympics for fair play, wherever you looked. Among coaches and athletes there was widespread suspicion that the Germans, both East and West, had received several hometown decisions. In one case, the American pole vaulters (including defending Olympic champion Bob Seagren) were told at the last minute that they would have to use the black poles favoured by some Europeans, rather than the newer green models, which rebounded differently and with which they'd competed all year. After Wolfgang Nordwig of East Germany parlayed this advantage into a gold medal, Seagren presented his substitute pole to Adrian Paulen, the president of the International Amateur Athletic Federation—and suggested where Paulen might place it.

In another incident, the West German Klaus Wolfermann led in the javelin to the very last throw, when Janis Lusis, the Soviet world record holder, uncorked a beauty. It appeared to be a winner until the Olympic officials declared that the Soviet's heave had fallen two centimetres short.

Most disturbingly, Vince Matthews and Wayne Collett, the Americans who had finished one-two in the 400 metres, were disqualified by IOC officials from the upcoming 1,600-metre relay after they stood casually—rather than at attention—as their anthem played during their award ceremony. The Americans, the overwhelming favourites going in, now had too few runners to compete, making the West Germans the best bet for the gold medal. But after leading the relay in the stretch, the home team faltered and failed to place.

The ultimate outrage—the one that would come to symbolize these troubled Games—occurred outside of competition. Security in the Village was a joke. During the day, the rear gate was manned by a single guard, who locked the gate at night and went home. Latecomers simply hopped the six-foot, chain-link fence to avoid the long walk around the perimeter to the front gate. Even when the guard was present, virtually anyone could get inside. I knew several Canadians who manufactured their own passes by laminating their photo onto an actual-size sample pass in the official press booklet. (A bogus pass could get you free meals, free admission into the stadium, and a free place to sleep, even if it was only the floor of a friend's room.) Others borrowed a team member's official jacket, and the guard would wave them through without checking.

In the pre-dawn of September 5th, eight Black September terrorists crept into the Village, killed two Israeli team members, and took nine others hostage in a dormitory at 31 Connollystrasse—just two buildings and 50 yards away from the Canadian team. (Like most of the third-string countries, we were clustered at the remote end of the Village, far from the television lounges and massage rooms reserved for the top dogs.)

As the tense day wore on, we watched the besieged building from our corner stairwell. A huge crowd gathered outside the fence, carrying signs like, "Make Sport, Not War." Meanwhile, we could see German soldiers shuttling into the Village to an assembly point behind the Koreans' building next door. They were thinly disguised in Puma sweat suits, and carried matching bags which contained their helmets and machine guns.

We were told to keep our heads down at 5:00 P.M., when the soldiers were scheduled to storm the Israelis' building. At 4:30 the police tried discreetly to push the crowd away from the fence. But the people refused to move and the rescue plan had to be abandoned, as it would have been all too easy for the terrorists to flip a few grenades over the fence or to spray bullets into the crowd with their AK-47s.

That night the terrorists and their hostages were ferried to the Munich Airport by helicopter. Shortly after landing, West German snipers opened fire, and the rest is history: nine more Israelis died, along with five Palestinians and one policeman.

(Back in the Village that night, there was a morbid footnote. After climbing a pole to steal a souvenir flag, an athlete lost his grip and fell to his death.)

The massacre evoked little outward emotion among the Village survivors. The incident was jolting, even numbing—but there were still races to be won, medals to be earned. Olympic athletes are the most single-minded people on earth. Their grand obsession cannot be shaken by a last-minute intrusion of the real world.

The next afternoon I sought out Heinz Piotrowski, the former Canadian team physio who now worked for Adidas. He took time off to treat my injured upper thigh, which had turned several shades of purple. As Heinz examined me, Lionel Pugh stopped by and saw the bruise; he must have concluded that my injury was for real. "Yesterday's events make our own problems pale into insignificance," he said, in a conciliatory gesture.

He was right, of course, but I'd already put my Olympics into perspective. Granted, I'd caught some bad breaks, but I knew that excuses were moot. No matter where you finished, that was your place—end of story. The finality lay especially heavy at the Olympics, since most people never got a second shot.

In retrospect, I realized that my chosen sport was one of ultimate frustration for almost everyone who played. There can be only one Olympic champion. The rest of us must confront our limitations. It might happen at the local level, or at the national, but we reach a point where we stop winning. (The purest expression of competitive agony is the face of a silver medallist just after a near-miss for the gold. *I've lost*, the face tells you. *I'm a loser*.) I'd thought I'd hit that wall two years earlier, a fact which tempered my disappointment in Munich. Percy had given me a second athletic life, and for that I was grateful.

Back in Toronto, my mentor offered a brief post-mortem: "We went a long way with the cards that were dealt us." It was pointless to wonder what might have been. I was reminded of my old first-grade running mate, Jack Robbins, whom I'd met socially after running my 10.1. After the obligatory exchanges, Robbins blurted out: "Yeah, I should have stayed with track—I was beating you before." In his mind, his relative prowess at age six would have been repeated at any level, had he only tried.

Transition

At 22 years old, the typical male athlete is quickest in his reflexes. At 30, he peaks in strength. Assuming he has adequate training and remains free of serious injury, he should record his best performances between those ages.

But by early 1973, at the age of 24, my perennial strains and pulls were catching up to me, and I knew it was time to start moving on—to make a living, for starters. I took a job as an insurance underwriter. I kept in touch with Percy, but there was no time to work with him as I had before. I trained around my job the best I could; I ran up and down stairs in my apartment building and spent some evenings at the University of Toronto, my nominal club at the time. Our indoor facility was a grim affair, housed in the South Industries Building at the Canadian National Exhibition grounds. We called it the Pig Palace—because it often hosted livestock shows and smelled heavily of animal urine. The track was a rather hazardous amalgam: a rubber surface, laid down in strips, over banked wooden turns and concrete straightaways. The rubber strips tended to draw back upon themselves, leaving small gaps of concrete in between.

I was drifting through the winter when Heinz Piotrowski, the ex-physiotherapist, told me that Gerard Mach had agreed to become Canada's national sprint coach. While he wouldn't work directly with any runners, Mach would consult closely with our other coaches, attempt to improve their techniques, and help plan our top athletes' programs. Mach, Heinz asserted, was "the best in the world." He had taken charge of his native Poland's sprint team in 1959. Seven years later, at the European Championships, Mach's athletes made a clean sweep of all 10 sprint events. His top star, Irena Szewinska, won the gold medal in the 200 at the 1968 Olympics and set the world record several times. Mach's specialty was the 400 metres, but he knew his business in the shorter sprints as well. There was a famous story in track circles about a British sprinter named Walter Manning, a good starter who always died at the finish and had never run better than 10.8 in the 100 metres. Manning's family was Polish, and in 1963 he moved to Poland— changing his name back to Wieslaw Maniak—to train with Mach. A year later, Maniak finished fourth at the Tokyo Olympics in 10.4.

The CTFA had lured Mach across the ocean out of a growing desperation, the fear that Canada would be humiliated at the 1976 Summer Olympics to be held in Montreal. It was a quick fix, but it might have worked had Mach been given the support he needed to run a world-class program. In fact, the low-budget status quo prevailed; our track and field program was hamstrung by Sport Canada, the government funding agency which subsidized and monitored the nation's amateur sports through its accredited organizations, from Judo Canada and the Federation of Canadian Archers to the Canadian Track and Field Association. From its inception in 1969, Sport Canada was a classic bureaucracy, insulated from the coaches and athletes it was designed to serve.

(At an international track coaching conference in Europe in 1973, each participant described his or her country's mode of administration. "We have a wheel system," the Soviet representative explained, "where the most promising athletes are fed to the best coaches at the centre." "We use the pyramid system," the East German delegate said, "in which the best athletes are moved to the top." When the floor passed to Lynn Davies, the CTFA's newly appointed technical director, he remarked, "Canada has the mushroom system—keep the athletes in the dark and dump crap all over them.")

Gerard was rudely awakened when he first called his runners together in May of 1973, to begin organizing his relay teams—his best hope, in the absence of any one outstanding talent, for a medal in Montreal. "We'll meet at the track at Etobicoke," he told me over the phone, in his thick accent. "I hear it's very good." When I arrived there, I found a stocky, balding man with extravagant grey muttonchops—and in a state of distinct agitation. The Etobicoke track is Grasstex, a reddish tar that is decent enough in dry weather, though not equal to the more modern Tartan, a synthetic rubber surface. But the track had been freshly coated, and on this moist Toronto spring day you could see pools of oil collecting on the surface. When we tried to get into a set position, our fingers slid uncontrollably.

"This is *garbage*," Gerard snapped. "Where is the nearest Tartan track?" We advised him that it was in Winnipeg—1,500 miles away. "My God!" said the new coach. "There are 100 Tartan tracks in Africa—we have six in Warsaw alone." He thought a minute and said: "Never mind, I know what we'll do. We'll go to Font Romeau in the French Pyrénées—they have a fantastic training centre at 7,000 feet. You're a rich country; we'll all go for six weeks. Then everything will be fine."

"Gerard," I said, "I can't go."

"What do you mean?"

"Well, I have to work."

"But, Charlie, you are the national champion—your company must send you and pay you, too."

It was apparent to me that Gerard had been sold a bill of goods by Canadian officials. He had no idea that track and field—an international passion and the core of the Olympics—was a neglected step-child in Canada. Gerard was dumbfounded when he discovered that not only were our top senior sprinters unable to train full time (as did his athletes in Poland), but there was no money in our budget to take them to a training camp. Even worse, the CTFA had scheduled but two sets of competitions that year: the Pacific Conference Games in May and the national championships in September, with nothing in between.

Years later, I cornered Gerard after he'd had a few beers and said, "Look, nobody's ever asked how you did it in Poland. How did you build that sprint group?"

And he said, "All right, you want to know? By 1966, I had a million U.S. dollars for the sprint section of my club alone. [Adjusting for inflation, that was about 10 times the competitive budget for the entire CTFA.] Plus I had unlimited resources within Poland. I put an ad in the Warsaw newspaper that said, 'Gerard Mach will audition sprinters,' and I got a *thousand* people to show up at the try-out. And out of the thousand, after a couple weeks of camps and tests, I chose the top hundred. And I took the whole hundred to an altitude training camp in Bulgaria and I kept them in training for six weeks.

"If I left the Eastern Bloc, and Western money was needed, the federation might cut me back a little—I was only allowed to take 70 sprinters to Formia, in Italy. But I had competitions, training camps, facilities—everything I needed."

There was a special brand of toughness to Gerard Mach. I wouldn't have blamed him if he'd turned around and gone back to where they took his sport seriously. But I would learn that the man had no breaking point—that he would fight for any scrap he could get.

In Canada, he had met his match.

At the outset that summer, I was in such poor shape that I could hardly run at all, and lost local races to people I'd always beaten. I improved with warmer weather, but my abbreviated training had left me far behind my rivals, too far to catch up in time for the 1973 nationals.

It was then that I decided to see if steroids would help me.

In truth, my mind had been made up at Munich. The question wasn't especially complicated. There was no risk of detection or disqualification, since steroids were not yet banned. I harboured some mild concern about health risks, and so I consulted my *Compendium of Pharmaceuticals* at work. The text warned of Dianabol's potential side effects, ranging from nausea to impotence. The warning was mild by comparison, however, to that attached to other steroids like Anadrol-50, which had been linked to liver damage. The risk seemed small and unproven, and the benefit substantial.

It all boiled down to one issue: Did steroids work as well as the athletes in Munich had claimed? The official line from Sport Canada was that anabolics were useless—but I'd learned to distrust the official line.

On the other side there was my intelligence from Brian Donnelly, a friend and retired Canadian hurdler who'd discussed steroids with a Soviet thrower. The thrower had confided that he was on a regimen of 35 milligrams of Dianabol per day—and that Valery Borzov, who had trained with him in the late 1960s, had been in the same drug protocol. (Years later, Donnelly's disclosure about Borzov's drug use would be confirmed to me by Valentin Chumak, the former Soviet hammer thrower, who'd also been in Borzov's junior development group.)

I also pored over the medical literature. A Soviet study on rats concluded that Dianabol achieved its maximum effect at a dose of .5 milligrams per kilogram of body weight—numbers which roughly conformed to the amounts reportedly taken by the Soviet thrower and Borzov. A 1971 American study found decisive strength benefits from Dianabol taken in 10-milligram doses. But in a double-blind study at Leeds University in England, where the Dianabol and placebo groups were asked to perform the same training tasks, *100*-milligram doses failed to result in any strength gains. As I weighed this report against the other data, it became clear to me that steroids were no magic potion. They worked only if combined with the right training, and if the athlete did *more* work—in either quantity or quality—than before.

Three weeks before the nationals I went to my family physician, explained what I was after, and asked for a prescription. My doctor expected no side effects with Dianabol. He prescribed 5 milligrams per day, the *Compendium*'s recommended therapeutic dose, which sounded right to me for an initial trial.

I used the Dianabol straight through the national championships—a less than optimal program, I'd learn later, but effective nonetheless. I soon began feeling less fatigued in training, able to push myself further without strain. I saw clear gains in muscle mass, yet lost several pounds of fat. Subjectively, I felt cheerful and positive. Four days before the big race I ran a 10.3 in a minor meet—my best showing since I'd become a part-time athlete. I went out to Vancouver and won the nationals easily.

Graduate School

If Percy Duncan gave me my first real education in sprinting, Gerard Mach provided a master's course. Gerard's English was poor; when he lectured groups of athletes, the kids would put on their earphones and tune him out. And because he was careful to avoid any appearance of poaching on other coaches' turf, I had to pursue him for advice. But if you asked the right questions, Gerard was a tremendous resource—a brilliant person in his field. Not everything he said made sense to me at first, but I was ready to consider it. When a coach produced top-level athletes as consistently as Gerard had, he had to be doing something right.

Gerard was the first coach I'd known to differentiate between muscular fatigue and central nervous system fatigue. In his view, the muscles were affected by both high- and low-intensity training, but they also bounced back quickly, within 24 hours. The central nervous system, by contrast, was affected primarily by high-intensity work (maximum or near-maximum-speed sprinting or heavy weightlifting), but it also required more time to recover, a full 48 hours.

The concept was simple enough, but it had revolutionary implications in North America, where the vast majority of sprinters laboured in a chronic state of nervous system exhaustion. They displayed, as I had at Stanford, all the telltale symptoms: flickering eyelids, twitching muscles, cramps, sleeplessness, irritability. Because of this syndrome, American runners often ran their best immediately after an injury, when they'd been forced to take some overdue rest.

Gerard understood that the only way to keep runners fresh—and able to run their best, in both training and competition—was to schedule speed work every *other* day. (Taking this principle further, Gerard would prescribe *10 days* of rest from speed work to recharge an overtrained runner. The fatigued athlete would maintain fitness with daily bouts of slower-tempo running and calisthenics.)

As Gerard settled into his new job, coaches would usher their young prodigies to him and ask the master for guidance. Billy's 12 years old, they would say, and he wants to run the 200 metres, so what should I do with him today, tomorrow, the next day? More often than not Gerard would reply, "I don't know," to the distress of his would-be disciples. Gerard shied away from dictating work assignments unless he knew all the variables at play. In training, no one size could fit all. How strong was Billy? How many years had he trained? What were his deficiencies?

Gerard's greatest influence on my own future coaching lay in his programming: his ability to construct an annual plan of training and competitions for athletes to run their best when it counted most, and to progress from one year to the next. This might sound like simple common sense, but in North America it was rarely practised. The United States could succeed through trial and error because it overwhelmed the world with sheer numbers. If you have thousands of sprinters on college scholarships, ten are bound to develop into good ones no matter *how* they're trained, and one or two of those will peak precisely at the World Championships or the Olympics. But Canada confronted these legions with a single platoon. At most, we might support 20 sprinters with minimal government subsidies. We couldn't afford to waste a single one.

(According to a Sport Canada policy born in 1973, these subsidized competitors—known as "carded" athletes—were classified according to their best performances of the past year: A-cards went to athletes ranking among the top 8 in the world in their event; B-cards to those among the top 16; and C-cards to those among the top 50, or for less developed athletes with strong potential. At the time, all carded athletes received $250 a month. These stipends were later raised to $650 a month for A-cards, $550 a month for B-cards, and $450 a month for C-cards.)

Gerard believed in "double periodization," with two distinct segments: a winter indoor season and a summer outdoor season. Within each segment there were three phases: a preparatory phase, a main work phase, and a competition phase, each of which emphasized different training components and varied the proportion of work to rest. Without periodization, an athlete works at the same level year-round and inevitably grows stale, since he will stop improving after six to eight weeks at a given task. Gerard understood the need to vary the stress on the organism—to increase the work demand, or cut it, or shift to a different component—if you wanted to keep expanding an athlete's capacity.

Gerard had been a bear about such details in Poland, and he tried to instill the same meticulous approach in Canada. He was dismayed to find resistance in his adopted country's track world— to his ideas, and to the extra effort they would entail. He was confronted with the mumbo-jumbo then making the rounds among Canadian coaches: that runners must be psychologically strong, above all else, to win at the top. Exhibit A was Valery Borzov, whose success in Munich was attributed to hypnosis. As the story went, Borzov had raised his hands in triumph after winning both the 100 and 200 metres. Then, after running the final leg in the Soviets' 4x100 relay team in a *losing* performance, Borzov raised his hands a third time—a programmed response, according to the theory.

In fact, the Soviet relay team had overachieved by winning the silver with only two top runners—a feat that Borzov naturally celebrated with his gesture. In Munich he had been a man among boys, for he *knew* that no one could touch him. (He set sea-level world records in both the 100 and 200 despite easing off at the end in both events.) He didn't get his confidence from a psychologist's couch. He got it from being physically ready.

At the 1976 Olympics, Borzov finished a disappointing third in the 100 metres after being injured beforehand. The Russian held second place late in the race behind Hasely Crawford, but began struggling to catch the leader and tightened up, allowing Don Quarrie to pass him on the other side. "Where was the hypnosis then?" Gerard would ask. "When you're prepared you can do whatever you want, but when you're not prepared you'll run like a beginner. Preparation is number one, number two, number three, number four, number five, number six—and when you get to number 97, we'll talk about psychology."

In the summer of 1974 Gerard arranged a European tour for our national team, the athletes who represent Canada in international competition. (The trip was subsidized by the newly created Sport Canada.) My physical problems had worsened, and I could run no better than 10.5, but I decided to make the best of it and enjoy myself. The highlight was our stay at the Polish national training centre in Warsaw, the Stadium Skra—Gerard's old stomping grounds. The stadium was heaven for an athlete, a place where utility was all. Our dorm rooms, for example, had been constructed under the second-level stands. In the morning we'd get up, go for breakfast at a stadium cafeteria, work out on the track, return to our rooms for a nap, and go back out for more work—as often as we wanted.

We also saw how much stature Gerard retained in Poland, as the nation's press gathered in his room each night. One day Gerard strolled into the cafeteria and asked us how we liked the food. I said that the food was fine, but that we had wearied of mineral water and wanted some Coca-Cola. He made a single phone call—and twenty minutes later a truck arrived and dropped off 80 *cases* of Coke. This explained why Gerard couldn't understand Canada's sluggish bureaucracy; he'd never had to deal with one before. In Poland, bureaucrats had been assigned to fulfill his wishes, rather than impede them. When Gerard wanted to take people to a training camp, he'd simply say the word—and the next day he had the visas, the plane tickets, the spending money in hand. He never had to run bake-athons or bingos. He made people run faster, and that was enough.

I spent my spare time with the team's throwers, among them shot-putter Bishop Dolegiewicz and discus thrower Ain Roost, who loved to rib one another about their steroid consumption. All of the throwers claimed they were taking less than their teammates, but it was mostly a big joke, and everyone recognized that drugs were an essential part of their game. In England we heard the British shot-put champion, Geoff Capes, tell us he'd taken to feeding Dianabol tablets to his parakeet. He'd tried to teach his musclebound bird to say, "Polly want a cracker—*now*."

Back in Canada, the next 18 months passed unremarkably. Each weekday morning I donned my jacket and tie and went to work. Each evening I would throw on my sweats and work out. But I knew my running career was over, and my training was dispirited. My favourite times were my talks with Gerard, when I'd pocket every nugget of information I could mine, or my informal sessions at the Pig Palace, when I'd advise younger sprinters about their technique.

I was not oblivious to the irony of my circumstances. The more I learned, the less I was able to use that knowledge for myself. It was a contradiction with only one solution: a turn toward coaching.

And so in the spring of 1976, when Peter Cross of the Scarborough Optimists called me with an opportunity—no pay, no perks, no established talents—it was an offer I couldn't refuse.

A New Optimist

I knew all about the Optimists. They were the largest and most successful track club in Canada. They thrived because Ross Earl, the club's founder and driving force, was a man of surpassing dedication. Ross started the club as the East York Mercuries in 1961, and furnished its budget—about $120,000 a year by the late 1970s—from the revenues of bingo games that he ran four times a week. Where other clubs recruited individual athletes, Ross recruited the best coaches he could find and gave them free rein. Although Ross was based in the Toronto suburb of Scarborough, where he taught children with learning disabilities in the public schools, his club was necessarily decentralized, as it lacked a training facility of its own. The athletes worked out at the Pig Palace during the winter and at scattered high school tracks when the weather turned warm enough.

Peter Cross, the Optimists' resident sprint coach, was a wild man—a dynamic, hard-drinking former schoolteacher. He was also one of the better coaches around, the first to throw his lot in with Gerard and follow the Pole's lead, and one of the few in Canada to scour for talent in the inner cities. In May 1976, Peter was bound for a pre-Olympic training camp in Los Angeles with his senior sprinters. He had four other runners who had just joined the club and would need looking after, which is where I came in.

I'll never forget those four kids: Clovis Locke, Dave McKnight, Ray Daley, and Carl Brown. Clovis was 19, the other three only 16. Like most of those who would join me later, they came from poor West Indian families. New to the game, with no preconceptions, they were all eager to learn and improve. Unlike U.S. track clubs, which functioned as managerial and sponsorship enterprises for mature stars, Canadian clubs had no talent pool from the colleges to draw on, nor even a formal feeder network from the high schools. Membership was open to any young athlete, regardless of ability, who displayed enough interest to come out on a regular basis. If they showed up, we took them in. I found that this policy suited me—that the most satisfying part of my job lay in developing people from scratch. The day a coach closes his door to new hopefuls is the day he starts planning his retirement; no matter how good they are, no stars last forever.

I was readily accepted by my young charges, in part because of my reputation as a former national champion. When you're 16 years old and running 11-flat, a 10.1 sounds impressive. I was still fit enough at 27 to train with my athletes, a great help in building rapport. I also picked up their patois, which would enable me to share their rowdy stories over the years.

I'd run practice from 5:00 till 7:30 four evenings a week, and for another two hours on Saturday afternoons. We'd start with some of Gerard's drills, for both warm-ups and fundamentals, and then alternate sessions of speed work with tempo work.

As resources were in short supply, we improvised. We had no starting blocks, but I didn't want them yet, anyway. In competition, blocks are essential to hold one's feet at a 45-degree angle to the track, allowing the athlete to push off in the direction he wants to go—forward—with a minimum of wasted motion. But a premature focus on starts is a prescription for failure, in both the short and the long terms. As young runners are too weak to extend their bodies properly as they drive out of the blocks, formal start training will ingrain poor mechanics, and the runners will be saddled with failure at each session. By the time they gain enough power to use the blocks effectively, they'll need to unlearn their mechanical errors and overcome the anxiety that errors create.

Both Percy and Gerard had approached technical problems by isolating each component within a single drill, rather than attempting to correct mistakes in the actual running. In the same spirit, I devised a new array of exercises to improve my runners' starting skills outside the blocks, without their being aware of our goal. In one drill I had them lie on their stomachs (or their backs, or their sides), with their hands beside their face and flat on the ground. On the command—"Go!"—they would scramble to their feet and start running. They'd do it over and over again; my mentors had taught me that repetition was the key to mastery.

The beauty of the drill was that it was *natural* to move into a good sprinting position within three strides. Starting and acceleration skills were developed without inhibition. The athletes weren't worried about technique because they were having fun. When ready for the blocks, they'd automatically assume a proper position—and feel relaxed and confident.

I took to coaching from the start, but considered it a hobby. I worked from day to day, with no great expectations. I still thought of myself as an insurance man and enjoyed the amenities that a steady paycheque afforded, not least my Aston Martin sports car.

My sprint group grew by word of mouth, and by the end of the summer I had 10 runners. Clovis Locke stood out. He was an especially co-operative kid who lived out in the sticks with an uncle and had to take two buses to get to practice. After ten weeks of formal training, Clovis entered the 100 metres at the Olympic trials in Montreal, stumbled at the start, yet came back to place fourth— ahead of several members of Canada's Olympic relay team. (He wasn't selected because it was too late for him to start practising with the squad.) He went on to win the national juniors in the 100, but Sport Canada refused to card him, a decision that I never understood. Clovis took a scholarship at East Tennessee State, suffered a series of injuries, returned to Toronto upon graduation, and is now an accountant. Later on I would encounter other young runners who'd been carded despite mediocre times and poor work habits. As they squandered their opportunities I'd think of Clovis, and remember the unfairness of it all.

I followed the 1976 Montreal Olympics on television and watched Canada's nightmare unfold: We became the first host nation for a Summer Games not to win a single gold medal. But Gerard's relay teams, with their polished stick work and modernized training methods, did better than expected. At the 1972 Olympics, Canada had entered only one of the four relay events. This time around, all four of our teams made the finals, and two of them finished fourth. Gerard had created a base of good performance, but the problem was the next step: to get beyond respectability in international competition, and to *win*.

Desai and Ben

By the spring of 1977, I had 15 people in my sprint group—and my first star. I stumbled upon Desai Williams after Ray Daley saw him run in April at the regional high school championships. After immigrating from St. Kitts, Desai had been a soccer player for Northview Collegiate, a Toronto high school, and came out for track—at the late age of 18—only after the school cancelled its soccer program. "You've got to see this kid," Ray told me, and in May he cajoled Desai into training with us.

As I watched the newcomer, I was first aware of Desai's un-orthodox running style. He had very large hamstrings and small quadriceps (it usually went the other way around) and a loping stride which swung his legs high behind him, more like a 400-metre runner's. At first he ran alone, and I didn't think that he was going all that fast. It was only after he raced against my other runners that I saw just how well Desai could move.

His success came quickly. In seven weeks, he improved from a hand-timed 10.8 in the 100 metres to a 10.52 electronic (equivalent to a hand-timed 10.3) and won four gold medals at the Canada Games, a competition for developing athletes who were neither carded nor members of the national team. Later that summer he won both the 100 and the 200 sprints at the national junior championships, and did the same at a junior triangular meet in Los Angeles against the U.S. and Japan. After four months in the sport, he was one of the top teenaged sprinters in the world.

For all of his obvious talent, Desai would remain an enigma to me. You could joke with him at first meeting—he could be terrifically entertaining and funny—yet never get to know him. He was reluctant to voice any unhappiness or disagreement and would show his displeasure in more subtle ways—by not showing up for a work-out, for example. Even when all was well, he couldn't always make it to practice, since he lived twenty miles away. He'd compensate by running hills near his home and forget to call me to let me know. These were relatively small annoyances, however, and the CTFA carded Desai after he met the Olympic qualifying standard set by the IAAF. He was also my first male athlete to make the national team.

A month after Desai arrived, Ben Johnson launched his Optimist career in a less auspicious fashion. His older brother, Eddie, had begun working out with us the previous October. Eddie was a dedicated runner and a great raconteur, but he seemed too short—about five-four at the age of 18—to succeed at sprinting. Then, one day in May, Eddie coaxed Ben into coming along to a work-out at Lawrence Park Collegiate, a local high school. (Ben had come to Canada just the year before, joining his mother and five siblings in a two-bedroom apartment in a poor working-class suburb of Toronto.) I can't say that Ben bowled me over. At 15, he was at the ideal age to begin training, but he looked more like 12: a skinny, awkward kid of 93 pounds. He wore tattered, black, high-top sneakers that seemed too heavy for his long, pipe-stem legs. He *looked* slow, and he ran even slower than he looked. After a half-circuit around the track, he flopped down in the stands. I came over and asked him what was wrong. "F-foot weak, mon—gotta rest," Ben told me, in his thick Jamaican accent. (In patois, "foot" refers to any part of the body between the hip and the ground.) Like his brother Eddie, Ben had a noticeable stutter. He later told me he had acquired it after years of mocking his brother's impediment—until he found he couldn't stop.

Ben's stutter aggravated the language difficulties that confronted many children who moved from the Caribbean to Canada. He attended a high school that offered no college preparatory programs and seemed to expect little from its students. One of Ben's teachers, a young woman who had yet to lose her enthusiasm, called me to voice her concern for him. "Ben has more potential than most of the kids," she told me, "but the school's just not challenging him." But when I tried to arrange a transfer for Ben to another school, the principal seemed indifferent. He pointed to Ben's poor grades and reading test scores, as if a few numbers told him all he needed to know.

There must have been times when Ben was bewildered by his new culture. One day he visited a Toronto park with a few friends. It was lunchtime, and the boys had no food. So they did what hungry people did in Jamaica: They took out their sling-shots, shot down a few of the local birds (pigeons, in this instance), started a fire, and began roasting their prey for lunch. Unfortunately, the feast was broken up by local police.

Ben was the youngest kid in our club, and at first he couldn't beat anybody. (Back home in Jamaica, in the depressed port town of Falmouth, he'd been cut from his local track team three times.) But he refused to be discouraged, and showed up every day. His status began to change after Dave McKnight gave him a pair of used spikes. Once liberated from those high-top anchors, Ben became a different runner. A few days later he won his first official race, in the midget-age class. The competition wasn't tough—the kid who finished second was nicknamed Fudgie, for obvious reasons— but Ben was on his way. A month later, one of my older kids called to tell me he was quitting. "Now everyone's beating me," he complained, "*even Ben.*"

I still didn't think much of Ben's track future at that point. He was only five-foot-three, and I figured that he wouldn't get much taller than his brother. I didn't know that Ben's father, back in Jamaica, was six feet tall, nor that Ben would grow to 5-10 3/4. Nor that those big eyes of his were fixed on goals beyond my vision at the time.

As an athlete, I'd always known that sprinting was more complicated than it looked from the stands. As a coach, I found intricacies that I hadn't even guessed at. The 100 metres is track's ultimate challenge precisely because it is so austere, so *short*. The shorter the distance, the less endurance becomes a factor—and the less you can improve by dint of hard work. Precision matters more than effort. Since 100-metre runners travel faster than athletes in any other event, they are more sensitive to mistakes, from technical flaws to overtraining. Because their extreme speed puts so much strain on their muscles and tendons, there is less margin for error and a higher frequency of disaster; sprinters are highly vulnerable to injury even when handled well.

At the same time, the 100 resists progress—much less a breakthrough—like no other event. Every engineer knows that it is harder to refine a pen than a tractor. By the same token, it is more difficult to set new records in the 100 than in longer events. With all the obvious fat shaved long ago, a coach must wrestle with the sparest of margins.

In the greater athletic community, however, sprinters get little respect. Distance runners disdain them for their lack of suffering. These Calvinists equate pain with achievement and cannot imagine the stress of running so fast; they can't identify with what they can't do. Others presume that any event that lasts 10 seconds requires sheer talent (true enough) and nothing more (a great miscalculation). I once met Jack Donahue, Canada's national basketball coach. "Sprint coach—what a tough job," he said. " 'Run fast; turn left.' " This attitude was common outside the discipline.

In fact, sprint coaching is a craft of constant adjustments and interconnected variables, as became apparent during our 1977 season. When I realized my runners were fatigued by our volume of speed work, I cut back from the year before—from three times to twice a week, with a weekly total of 1,500 metres, a little less than a mile. To further reduce the stress on my sprinters' central nervous systems, I shifted some of their speed volume from short sprints to weekly "special endurance" runs, from 150 to 300 metres.

I conducted all speed work at 100 percent of my runners' capacity—and since my runners always had adequate recovery periods between work-outs, their capacity was consistently high. My theory was simple: Sprinters needed to train at race pace, both to imprint the higher speeds on their muscle memory and to acclimatize their muscles and tendons to the demands of racing. My athletes would run only two special endurance segments once a week and would rest up to a half-hour between the two, but I asked them to go absolutely all out every step of the way. (They were pleased to oblige. Nothing makes a sprinter happier than going as fast as he can—especially if he's feeling rested.) I cared only about the quality of the runs. The quantity was almost irrelevant.

To reduce the risk of injury, I regularly massaged my sprinters, especially before their speed work. By loosening their muscles, massage enhanced their performance and removed lactic acid and other fatigue by-products from their muscles. Massage also gave me an added safety check. None of my kids ever wanted to skip a speed run. If I asked if they felt tight, they'd deny it. But their muscles couldn't lie, and a massage often clued me to pull an athlete out of a run *before* something went wrong.

No one in North America conducted special endurance drills this fast. Not Gerard, who worried that athletes might be injured if they exceeded 95 percent of their maximum in training (and thus deferred the risk to the time of competition). Not the American coaches, who entered their people in too many meets to permit maximum-speed runs in practice. And not my fellow Canadian coaches, who prescribed excessive volumes and truncated recovery cycles. Even if their athletes survived the gruelling work-outs, they could never fulfill their potential as runners, since they would always be fatigued from the work of the day or the hour before. Come the meets, they would be accelerating with their brakes on.

I didn't broadcast my heresy, and I was nervous when Gerard finally took in one of our special endurance sessions. I was afraid he might throw a fit once he saw how fast we went. The first runner to go was one of Peter's kids: Hugh Spooner, a 1976 Olympian. From a running start, he ran 300 metres in a smooth 35.9. "Very nice," Gerard nodded. Then Angella went out—and ran 35.8. "Jesus!" Gerard exclaimed. Then it was Desai's turn. After lining up with Brian Saunders, the Canadian 400-metre record holder, Desai flew through the mark and hit the 200-metre split in 19.7, a world-record pace. Though he tailed off toward the end, he finished in 31.6—leaving Saunders 25 metres in his wake.

Gerard was agog. "No wonder these people are running so fast in the meets," he said. "All they have to do is repeat their practice times!" He never raised the matter again.

My people were putting the sprint establishment on notice. In June of 1977, a Canadian Olympic coach offered to drive a vanload of my kids to a race in Montreal. I sent six sprinters, including Desai, Eddie Johnson, Ray Daley, and Dave McKnight. On the way, the coach sang the praises of the favourite in the 100 metres that day, a kid named Dan Biocci who had made the Olympic team the year before. "There's no way you'll beat him," he warned my group, "but you can aim at the other guys."

As it turned out, all six of my sprinters made the 100-metre final, and this is the way they finished: 1-2-3-4-5-6. Biocci ran seventh.

Tony, Mark, and Angella

When my group resumed training in the fall of 1977, I found myself surrounded by 30 young athletes. I hadn't sought the new ones out; they simply presented themselves at the track. While I knew I'd be facing more headaches in the year to come, I welcomed the influx. Coaches need a big enough group to give their system a chance, to ensure that they'll have enough raw talent to draw from.

This principle cuts both ways; the more athletes you have, the fewer excuses. "Look," Gerard would tell me, "if you coach a large enough cross-section of athletes, and you don't have a single athlete who can run 10.5 in the 100 metres, you *can't* be doing the right things. To go below that you need to get some natural talent—maybe you will, maybe you won't. But if you've been coaching 10 years, and your guys are all running 10.7, 10.8, 10.9, you're not a coach and your athletes should leave you—you're incompetent." His assessment was blunt but fair.

A sprint coach reaches a pivot point when he finds his first big talent. Many coaches might have seized upon a Desai Williams as the answer to their prayers, dumped their other runners, and spent all their time in grooming a single superstar. The problem is that there's no way of telling which teenager will turn out best—who will burn out, who will bloom late. Had I concentrated exclusively on Desai, I would have wound up with a good international runner but missed out on the ultimate. Instead, I'd kept the door open that spring for an unlikely-looking Ben Johnson, and it was still open in October, when Tony Sharpe and Mark McKoy came calling.

Where Ben had seemed younger than his years, Tony was a 15-year-old in a man's body—5-11 and 170 pounds, with muscular arms and an imposing physical presence. I liked him from the start. He was more easy-going than my other top runners, less demanding, impossible to stay mad at. He was also more advanced than any runner I'd known at his age; at a stage when Ben was running 11.1 in the 100 metres, Tony had been timed in 10.4. (He was precocious enough to be carded at the end of the season, two years before Ben.) Tony wasn't exactly maintenance-free, however. He was highly distractable, especially where women were concerned. He had a reputation as a ladies' man, and it got worse as word spread and the girls tried to warn off their friends—which only egged them on, of course.

(Gerard could sympathize with me on this score. He'd once set up a special meet to allow one of his European champions to take aim at a world's indoor record. Gerard plotted the runner's training schedule for weeks in advance, and everything appeared perfect—except that his star proceeded to run like a dog. "What happened?" Gerard demanded after the race. "I'm sorry, coach," the runner sheepishly replied, "but Miss Poland came to my room last night—what could I do?")

In those first months, Tony was motivated most by an ugly shirt. We handed out different-coloured singlets—the standard sleeveless track shirts—with the colours keyed to the athlete's best performance. At the top of the heap, those who had run 10.4 or better wore a revolting hue of orange. The shirts intimidated rival athletes, since word soon spread that any kid wearing orange was someone to be reckoned with. Tony asked for an orange shirt almost every day, but he'd always run his 10.4 at a minor meet that none of us had witnessed, so we kept holding out for more proof. It became a stock gag.

Mark McKoy was Tony's inseparable companion, so much so that we took to calling him "The Shadow." He was self-contained even as a 14-year-old. He simply went his own quiet way—until his lanky frame drew stares as it flew past people on the track. He never introduced himself to me, and for a long time I didn't know who he was, nor that he'd joined the club. (The state of the Optimists' paperwork ranged from bad to abysmal.) I was also unaware that Mark had been taught to hurdle by his previous coach, Bill Rashbrook, who'd put together an extraordinary group of midget-age (under 16) athletes.

The story of that group encapsulates both the fluky nature of track stardom and the negligence that riddles the sport. After Rashbrook quit coaching to salvage his family life, 10 of his athletes went to a nearby public high school and the other two to Senator O'Connor, a Catholic school. The public school kids were all ruined by overtraining on a hard terrazzo floor, which destroyed their ankles and knees. The two parochial school survivors were Tony and Mark—leaving us to imagine the talent that had been lost.

In Canada, as in most countries, men's and women's sprinting were segregated affairs. I'd never subscribed to that tradition. It seemed to me that sprinting was sprinting, assuming you ran upright and had two feet, and that individual variations were primary, regardless of gender. In January 1978, when three young women joined our group, I soon found I'd been right. If the women were different in any way, it was that they were more compliant in following instructions, but needed those instructions to be detailed and precise. I liked to give my sprinters options in training, but the women preferred a more structured style.

One of the three newcomers was Angella Taylor (later Issajenko), a 19-year-old who had been recruited by Peter Cross for my group of junior runners. He had found her at a high school meet at the Pig Palace, where she'd run a fast 400 metres on a *boys'* relay team. (Upon coming to us she had assumed she would be working with Peter, and at first felt disappointed to land with me.) Angella stood out straight away—a striking girl with long, straightened reddish-black hair and a bright red sweatsuit. She became even more noticeable when she tried to hide behind a pillar while the group did warm-up drills, then slid into the crowd for the rest of practice. This went on for several days, until I deduced the problem: She was too embarrassed to try the drills because she didn't know the routine. Angella Taylor, I would discover, was a perfectionist in all things.

Angella was an only child who grew up with her great-grandparents in the Jamaican countryside and later went to boarding school. She followed her mother to Toronto in 1975, and a year later made a name for herself by winning some of the local high school meets. But she had no training—she was simply showing up for the races. Her practice time was limited, as she worked after school at a nursing home. She could afford only one pair of shoes, an old Adidas model with removable spikes. She'd use them as flats for jogging, then screw the spikes back in for competitions.

For a time Angella seemed destined to become just another promising runner who would fall by the wayside. The summer before we met, she had joined Toronto's Michael Power Track Club, which had somehow ignored her. By the time she got to me she was 19 years old, and her training was four years behind schedule. She needed a coach and a friend, and I was glad to be both—we hit it off right away. I found Angella to be fiercely loyal and dead serious about developing her gift. She was the hardest worker I'd ever met in my life, a virtue so extreme that it would land us in trouble later on. She usually kept her ambition to herself, but occasionally it slipped out. After winning one high school meet, she surprised me with a quote in a local newspaper: "I want to be the best in the world." When her teammates poked fun at her lofty aspirations, she refused to back down. "What do you want me to try to be?" she demanded. "Should I try to be number two?"

While naturally fast, Angella was slightly overweight and lacked fitness. Her technique was adequate, however, and her loose stride promised better things to come. In her first race for us she ran 6.7 seconds in the 50 metres—no threat to the Canadian record, but more than enough to rout the high school kids she was up against.

Angella's biggest weakness was her starts, due mainly to her lack of strength, a problem we couldn't attack in earnest until the coming fall, after the season concluded. One day I asked Gerard to meet us at Etobicoke to watch Angella practise: I wanted to unveil my new talent. As first impressions go, it was a disaster. First Angella lost her gold anklet, and the three of us spent 15 minutes on our hands and knees on the Grasstex before we found it. Then she proceeded to start—and performed miserably, even by her standards. After a long silence, Gerard said, "Maybe the 400 metres—not the 100." Like others before him, he had written Angella off. And like the others, he couldn't have been more wrong.

The Pig Palace was available to us only until mid-March, leaving us to the mercy of Toronto's bleak spring weather and costing us valuable practice time. To help fill the gap, I proposed to van my runners to a 10-day spring training camp at East Tennessee State, where they could train indoors or out and spare their legs by running on grass, the best preventative measure against shin splints. Ross Earl agreed to raise $1,500 toward hotel costs, and I matched it with an advance on my credit card. According to club policy, each athlete was supposed to contribute $35 toward meals. To spare the kids embarrassment, I distributed empty envelopes to my runners and asked them to deposit whatever they could afford. Most of the envelopes came back empty, as I knew they would.

The camp exceeded expectations, especially for Angella, who lowered her best 200-metre special endurance time by a full second as soon as she stepped outdoors. Tony was also working well, but I never knew how Ben would run on a given day, even after he'd confirmed his promise the month before by running fourth—against grown men—in the 50 metres at the Canadian National Indoor Championships in Montreal. I attributed Ben's inconsistency, a pattern that would hold for the next two years, to his prodigious growth spurt. He had gained 40 pounds and grown six inches in the nine months I'd known him, approaching his full-grown height, and his appetite was alarming. I had a refrigerator in my motel room in Tennessee, and Ben came by every day to make half a dozen ham or roast beef sandwiches—his between-meals snack. On one occasion, he consumed an entire family barrel of Kentucky Fried Chicken and washed it down with a banana split. Ben's metabolism was on tilt, and his every other thought seemed to be of food. (The camp was much healthier for him than some previous expeditions. At a road stop for lunch during a February trip to a meet in Montreal, I watched Ben and his brother slowly study the menu and finally order a single plate of French fries, which they shared. When I asked them why they were eating so little, they explained they had only six dollars between them to last the three days.)

One morning in Tennessee we went to a diner for breakfast— Ben's first attempt at ordering at a restaurant.

"What ch'all want today?" the waitress drawled.

"*Heggs*," said Ben, with some urgency.

"How you like 'em?"

"*Lot!*" said Ben.

"Don't listen to him," said Eddie, who shut his brother up and took charge of the meal.

"Lord, that kid can *eat*," Eddie told us one day when Ben was out of the room. "One morning Ben got up before the rest of us and just cleaned the kitchen out. By the time we got up, there was absolutely nothing left in the house—not a pat of butter, not a stalk of celery, nothing. He ate *seven* breakfasts."

I found that Ben had other appetites, as well. I was relaxing with several athletes in my hotel room when a local girl dropped by to see Val Grose, a senior runner she'd met in a bar earlier that evening. "Say, Val," she said, "maybe I'll come by later—what room are you in?" From Val's reaction, it was apparent that he wasn't that interested. "Two-fourteen," he muttered, hoping she wouldn't hear.

"What was that?" she said.

"Two-sixteen!" Ben piped up, substituting his own room number.

After the girl left, Ben's roommate Mike Collymore (who later played in the Canadian Football League) began mocking the would-be Lothario. "Ben, you wouldn't know the first thing to do if that girl showed up," he said.

"Yah, mon," Ben countered.

"Okay, Ben, what's the first thing you do?"

Ben laughed and said: "T-t'row your ass out da door."

Fifty miles down the road, at the national team's camp in Knoxville, things weren't going so well. They had a rash of athlete injuries—most tragically that of Cindy Moore, the Canada Games champion in the 100 metres. Cindy had been forced to do single-leg jumps off a three-foot-high box, a dangerous exercise which she'd never done before. She broke her ankle and never fully recovered.

Even in his adolescence, a phase when most of us are desperate for outside approval, Ben judged everything by his own standards. He alone would determine his success or failure. A classic example came that June at the Black Heritage Meet at Lawrence Park, at which a sizeable portion of Toronto's black community annually turned out. Ben and Tony took on the neighbourhood speed kings in the juvenile division of the 100 metres. Predictably, the two of them cleared the rest of the field by 10 yards, and both finished with wind-aided 10.3s. I thought Ben had nipped his teammate at the tape. But the judges awarded the race to Tony, who was instantly mobbed by the crowd. I was reminded of the difference between first and second; Ben, who'd run equally well, might not have existed.

Ben walked over to me in the stands and said, "I thought I won that race." His tone was serious but unemotional.

"I thought you did, too," I said.

"Yeah, that's what I thought," Ben said—without a single word of complaint. Ben knew he'd won and that was all he cared about. I was fascinated by his response, and by the self-confidence that lay behind it.

Progress

That summer marked a great leap forward for my sprinters. Not only did they see places far removed from their everyday circuit of home, school, and track, but they got a glimpse of how good they might become in a bigger arena. Ross Earl raised an extra $35,000 to sponsor our 20 best male athletes in a series of meets in Switzerland and West Germany. Ben was in Jamaica to visit his father, a telephone lineman who'd been unable to find work in Canada and now lived apart from the family. But my group's other top men were with us, and their training suggested they were ready to do well. The trip's high point came at a dual meet against the Swiss national team in Aarau, near Zurich. The Swiss squad was slightly depleted, since a few of their better people were resting for the European Championships, but they were still counting on demolishing our kids. During one practice a Swiss coach walked up to me and said, "Who's your best sprinter?" I pointed to Desai, who was loping along with his odd stride. The coach inquired as to his personal bests, and I told him: 10.35 in the 100 metres and 20.99 in the 200. The Swiss coach was skeptical: "I'll have to see that."

On race day he saw it and then some. Desai popped a 10.31 (roughly equivalent to a hand-timed 10.1) in the 100, beating the nearest Swiss by three metres, and came back to win the 200, again by a huge margin, in 20.68. We couldn't keep pace with the Swiss in the distance events, but we swept the individual sprints and relays, and our throwers did well. At the final tally we'd scored a one-point upset, a tremendous psychological boost for us.

We had strong showings in the other meets as well, and by tour's end our athletes had totalled 22 new personal bests. That trip taught me a lesson I would never forget: That a coach must find the right level of competition to elicit top performances. We'd picked tough opponents, but not so tough that they would beat our kids into a coma. We'd had a legitimate chance to win, a far cry from the tradition at invitational meets back home, where a few outclassed Canadians were sacrificed for the sake of local interest. When unprepared athletes are thrown in against the best in the world, they panic. An athlete who was ordinarily capable of a 10.6 in the 100 might respond to the pressure by running a 10.9—a humiliating experience which might permanently scar his confidence.

At the 1978 nationals in Montreal, it became clear to all how much ground we had covered. With Peter Cross and me pooling our runners, the Optimists entered three squads—our seniors, juniors, and juveniles—in the 4x100 relays, the event which best measures a sprint program's depth. Our squads finished first, second, and fourth against the country's top provincial senior teams. Desai finished second to the senior Hugh Fraser in the 100. Angella placed second in the 200, only six months after she'd begun formal training. In the latter event, without any strength work, she had improved from 26.2 hand-timed to 23.81 electronic. Once she'd gotten into shape, her natural talent and hard work had pulled her ahead of the other women in our club—just as they would allow her, not so long thereafter, to surpass some of the biggest names in the world.

Despite Angella's dramatic improvement—and the strong likelihood that she'd reach 23-flat, the projected threshold for the Olympic finals in 1980—the CTFA's sprint coaches voted 10-2 that fall against carding her for the 1979 season. The loss of $250 a month would have been a cruel blow to someone as poor as Angella, except that Gerard ignored the consensus and successfully recommended her to Sport Canada for carding.

In little more than a year of part-time coaching, I had developed the dominant young sprint group in Canada, and one of the more promising squads in North America. Our progress was no fluke. Aside from our full-speed special endurance runs, I would attribute this success to five primary factors:

* *Letting my runners run.* My experience as an athlete definitely helped me here—not only in correcting mechanical flaws but in knowing when to leave well enough alone. Many technical glitches are symptoms of an underlying problem. For example, in 1978 a number of coaches criticized Angella's stride pattern—they felt she was over-striding. By the next year, the same people had reversed themselves: "Boy, you really fixed up her stride," they told me. In fact, I'd done absolutely nothing about it. After we improved her conditioning, her stride fell into place. Had we changed it in 1978, we would only have had to change it again, at the risk of spoiling her natural style.

When children run at play, they display instinctive form and rhythm. Most sprinters develop problems because someone wrongly corrected them, and they haven't been able to unlearn the correction.

Hands-on observation. The most brilliant training theories are useless if a coach fails to adapt them to each individual. Canned training schedules won't suffice. (I stopped using written workout instructions when I found my athletes treating them like some holy commandment for success, rather than a guide to be adjusted according to how they felt on a given day.) In distance running, oxygen uptake and lactic acid tests can help a coach keep track of his athletes' aerobic capacity. These tools are useless, however, for anaerobic events like sprinting; there is no machine to gauge central nervous system fatigue. My feedback came from my athletes, and so I'd constantly ask if they felt as if they needed to rest. But since mature athletes tend to ignore signs of fatigue and incipient injury—believing, as I used to, that *more* work is better—I couldn't always trust their responses. To protect them from themselves, I would listen to their footfalls during a drill. If the sound became louder, it told me the runner's hips were dropping. The drop might be as little as a sixteenth of an inch, beyond the discernment of eyes or cameras, but my ears would tell me that fatigue had set in, and that it was time to curtail the work-out.

* *Reinforcing the positive.* Young runners need all the moral support they can get. They are investing countless hours into an endeavour where the objective rewards—a medal, a ranking, carded status—may lie months or years down the road. To keep my runners enthusiastic about practising, I played to their strengths and picked my spots in offering criticism. Our special endurance runs were reserved for days when an athlete's immediate past form led me to expect improvement. At other times, the exercise would be varied to screen the runner from disappointment. I might change to a new distance (to prevent comparisons to past efforts), or direct the athlete to run "smooth" (at less than maximum speed). Or I might put the timer away.

* *Low-density coaching.* A basic coaching skill is to feed information in digestible amounts, to allow people to absorb the basics at their own rate. Many coaches are defeated by a compulsion to demonstrate their expertise and hence their authority. They overwhelm with peripheral detail and get impatient when their athletes become confused. By contrast, I might stress a single action for an entire work-out: the position of the left arm at the start, for example.

* *Patience.* In conducting technique drills (which included knee lifts, skipping, bounding, and hopping), most of my associates demanded perfect form, a sharp pace, and rapid retention. They produced quick studies but tight runners. I used the same drills, but paced them slow and easy—to keep my athletes relaxed, even though it took them longer to learn. In their own time, they would master all the required movements and be ready to transfer them to a race, without tension.

When my athletes were slower than usual in picking something up, I didn't keep pushing them. I read their dullness as central nervous system fatigue—a sign that they were insufficiently rested to learn—and promptly backed off. To do otherwise could be dangerous. Several years ago, a top-ranked pairs skating team kept missing the landing on a new throw manoeuvre. The more they tried, the worse it got. Rather than stopping them to resume another day, their coach asked for one more effort. They tried and failed again—and this time the woman skater sprained her ankle, costing the team an Olympic medal.

By the summer of 1978 it became apparent that my hobby had grown into something much larger. I wanted to see how far I could take this team—and so I quit my job, moved back with my parents, refinanced the Aston Martin to raise some living expenses, and began coaching full time. I knew there were no financial guarantees, but I didn't care. If it didn't work out after a few years, I figured the insurance industry would still be there.

Coaching was what I liked most and did best. I knew I'd entered a new phase when one of my young athletes paused during practice, looked at me curiously, and said, "You used to run, right?" It took me a moment before I was able to confirm the rumour. I'd become so involved with what I was doing that I'd blanked out my past life. I was a *coach* now.

Breakthroughs

In the fall of 1978, Peter Cross left Toronto to become an assistant sprint coach at Clemson University in South Carolina. He left with Desai Williams, Dave McKnight, and Ray Daley, all of whom accepted track scholarships there. I thought they would thrive with the superior climate and competition, and with a facility far superior to the Pig Palace.

Anxious to check in with Desai and the others, I brought 26 athletes down to Clemson in March 1979, for our warm-weather camp. The training was valuable but the scene was outrageous, culminating in a Clemson athlete totalling his car and throwing Dave McKnight through the windshield. Peter had promised us free use of a visitors' dormitory but hadn't cleared the deal with his athletic director. The director dropped by one morning and threw a fit when he saw our young women wrapped in towels at the ostensibly all-male dorm. The women were promptly ejected, forcing me to house them at a Holiday Inn and drain another $2,700 from my credit cards.

Soon I would begin to question Clemson's value. My athletes (including Tony and Mark, who had enrolled in January of that year) weren't improving, and I worried that they weren't getting enough speed work. They were bored and lonely, the chief local diversion being cow tipping (in which a student would sneak up on a standing, sleeping cow, then push her over). The final blow came early in 1980, when Tony slipped on some dormitory steps after a freak ice storm and tore the sheath of his Achilles tendon—an injury that would plague him for the rest of his career. By the end of that year, all of my sprinters had left Clemson for good, and Peter had beaten a retreat to the wilds of British Columbia.

Angella Taylor broke through in a big way during the 1979 indoor season. Her starts still handicapped her, but less than the year before, and she had so much speed that she could win even the shorter races. At the National Indoor Championships in Edmonton, she ran a total of seven heats and finals, in three events—the 50 metres, the 200 metres, and the 4x200-metre relay—and broke the Canadian record in all seven. She was approaching world-class times, and I knew she was ready when she left for Europe in late May with the national women's team.

Angella had barely disembarked from the plane in Italy before a sprint coach put her through a string of relay drills under the hot sun. (I was on a separate tour with the Canadian men's team at the time.) Tired from excessive practice, she ran 11.65 in her first meet—an official personal best, but far off her training times in Canada. Undeterred by his lack of familiarity with her program, the coach proceeded to alter Angella's start—he even switched her feet in the blocks! (This broke the cardinal rule for our national teams: *Never* tamper with another coach's athlete.)

The squad then travelled 24 hours by train to a dual meet on June 10th, 1979, in Karl Marx Stadt against the East Germans, the strongest team in the world. Our women arrived exhausted the day before the meet. The East Germans, meanwhile, were rested, prepared, and on their home turf. They broke three world records at that meet, and their 4x100 relay team beat the Canadians by more than three seconds. Angella strained her hamstring in the 100 metres and ran 11.69, far behind Marlies Göhr's 11.03 and Marita Koch's 11.12.

As Angella stood injured on the sidelines to watch the 200 metres, her strongest event, she became even more depressed. Her training times indicated that she could already perform in the 22.90 range. She was a full second faster than the year before, and it seemed reasonable to believe she could approach the 22-second level within two years. Marita Koch, who stood atop the 200-metre world list with a 22.06, had broken the record several times since 1977, but in relatively small increments, and might conceivably be overtaken. In Karl Marx Stadt, however, Koch broke the record again with a science-fictional 21.71—lopping off more than three tenths of a second in one blow.

Our targets were moving wildly now, and not just in Europe. At the U.S. Track and Field Championships a week later, Evelyn Ashford ran an improbable double of 10.97 (just nine hundredths off Marlies Göhr's world record in the 100) and 22.07. Ashford had dropped her personal best in the 100 metres by two tenths, spectacular enough, and in the 200 by *six* tenths. (Later that year, at the World Cup in Montreal, Ashford would lower her 200-metre time even further, to 21.83.) These prodigious gains were completely unexpected from an already world-ranked sprinter who had shown little progress over the previous three years. We'd entered a realm of statistical anarchy. Where might Koch and Ashford be going next?

Angella always kept tabs on her opposition, and she was shell-shocked. I had a month to repair her form and confidence before the Pan Am Games in Puerto Rico. The CTFA overlooked me for a coaching position, even though I trained every sprinter it selected for the Games—four men plus Angella. Ross Earl helped out with a round-trip plane ticket, and I went anyway. I regained control over my athletes and worked them carefully, with ample rest before the meet.

Going in, Angella's official personal bests were 11.64 and 23.59. At the Pan Ams, she ran the 100 in 11.41 in her heat, a wind-aided 11.26 in her semi-final, and 11.36 in the final—good enough for a bronze medal behind Evelyn Ashford and Brenda Moorhead, two established international stars. In the 200, Angella ran 23.13, 22.80, and 22.74—nearly a second below her personal best—and won the silver, again behind Ashford. I'd known from Angella's training times that she was ready to break through; had she been handled better in Europe, it might have happened six weeks earlier. The Pan Am Games represented our first great success at the world level.

But it would not be Angella's last word that season. At the Canadian Track and Field Championships, the annual national meet, she won both the 100 and 200—her first of 17 national outdoor sprint titles without a defeat. Desai matched her sweep on the men's side. Overall, I had seven of the eight finalists in the 100. My big three—Desai, Ben, and Tony—would go on to win 18 of the 19 national titles they would contest through 1988.

Finally, at the World Cup trials in Quebec City, Angella won with a new Canadian record of 11.20, and went on to place fifth in both the 100 and 200 at the Cup itself—a competition of eight regionally zoned teams from throughout the world—in Montreal. At the end of the 1979 season, less than two years after we'd begun her systematic training, *Track & Field News* ranked her tenth in the world in the 100 and ninth in the 200. (She was my first athlete to gain a world ranking, and would remain the only one until 1983, when Mark McKoy joined her. Ben would be ranked for the first time in 1984.) She had just turned 21, and was fast making up for her late start in the game.

The national men's team had travelled apart from the women in the summer of 1979, my first European tour as a coach. Ben wasn't yet on the team, since his best 100-metre time of 10.66 (as compared to Tony's 10.51 and Desai's 10.31) fell short of the standard. But the little-known 17-year-old had opened eyes at the Maple Leaf Indoor Games that winter in Toronto when he ran the 50-yard dash against a number of world-class senior sprinters, including Olympic champion Hasely Crawford. Ben was there strictly for the experience, but he surprised by advancing through the preliminary heats. As he lined up for the finals, I felt a spasm of protectiveness. Though Ben had grown to 150 pounds, his body still looked unformed, adolescent. While he didn't place in that race, he showed that he belonged. Gerard offered to pay half of Ben's expenses for Europe, and Ross and I covered the difference.

I didn't mind chipping in; in Canadian track, where government support was limited and the athletes tended to be poor, there was no practical alternative. And in Ben's case there was something more. Ben's mother, Gloria Johnson, was a cafeteria worker with six children. She'd taken a second job at night so that Ben could train without the interference of having to work after school. Just before we left for Europe, she gave me a hundred dollars to hold for Ben's spending money, and I knew what that sum must have meant to her. "Take care of him," she told me.

I did my best, although Ben's first transatlantic trip amounted to a series of mishaps. His on-track highlight came at a meet in Italy, when he was slotted to run the lead-off leg in the 4x100 relay against Pietro Mennea, by now a veteran European champion. Ben was thrilled about meeting one of the big guns in his sport, even after Mennea had trounced him.

In a more competitive setting, a 100-metre race against second-tier Polish and Italian athletes, Ben jumped out to an early lead—he'd established his trademark leaping start even then—in a torrential downpour. But while he could have beaten the other sprinters, he couldn't beat his own shirt. Our uniforms, cheap cotton singlets with oversized armholes, were truly awful. Their chief virtue was that they'd been supplied for free. Ben's shirt sopped up so much water that it began to droop, until it fell past his shoulders and bound his arms to his torso. By the last 10 metres he was virtually immobile, and the other runners glided past him. His teammates and I were in helpless hysterics on the sidelines, and Ben laughed as well. He realized that some things were beyond his control.

As the youngest member of our squad, Ben was a natural target for practical jokes. After a tri-meet with Britain and Kenya at Gateshead in northern England, we had a 5:00 A.M. wake-up the next day to begin a long trip to Italy. I told our athletes to go to bed early and to set their alarm watches, since they'd be rising before the sun. At midnight I was awakened by a clamour down the hotel corridor. There were my runners in their underwear, pointing and howling with glee. And there was Ben, standing fully dressed with his cap on, his bags packed, and a puzzled expression on his face. Some joker had moved Ben's alarm up five hours, and his teammates had been cued to watch the trap spring.

Decision

By the fall of 1979, my time had come to deal with the sport's great X-factor: anabolic steroids. While the IAAF had explicitly banned the drugs in 1975, the prohibition had been widely ignored. Testing was generally reserved for major international meets, although Britain's Amateur Athletics Association sometimes tested smaller meets as well. Even on those occasions, however, the procedure wasn't done by the book. The evening before our tri-meet with Britain and Kenya in Gateshead, meet officials called the team managers in to watch while they drew numbers out of a hat. Each number corresponded to a "place" for a given event. After a "3" was drawn for the 400 metres, for example, we knew they would test the third-place finisher—and him alone—in that race.

This advance notice blatantly contravened the IAAF's testing protocol, and its value became clear after we relayed the information to our athletes. Brian Saunders, who had been training with me that summer and was scheduled to run the 400, was upset. He'd been taking steroid injections and had been sloppy about it; he couldn't remember the date of his last shot or even the specific drug he'd used. "Look," I told him, "you better make sure that you don't finish third tomorrow." Saunders took my advice to heart. Late in the race he was neck and neck for second with a British runner. Finally, sensing that he wasn't going to win the duel, Saunders slowed to a jog. A Kenyan runner made up 15 metres and out-leaned him at the tape, and Saunders finished fourth—and safe.

None of my men was yet advanced enough to make steroid use an issue. Angella Taylor, however, was another matter. About to be world-ranked and still rapidly improving, she seemed poised to move to the very top. While I knew that steroids were commonplace at that level, Angella had been coming along so well without them that I'd been able to avoid the issue. But now we had to take another look. Our goal—a medal at the 1980 Olympics in Moscow—was hurtling away from us.

Numbers define one's place in the track world. Now our place was receding—and I felt sure I knew why. Angella wasn't losing ground because of a talent gap. She was losing because of a drug gap, and it was widening by the day. From what I saw and heard, it was clear that world-ranked women were using banned substances. As I tracked the steroid trail—the network of coaches, doctors, and managers known to be involved with drugs—I found that it led to athlete after athlete. I arrived at a central premise which would guide my counsel for Angella, as well as for Ben and my other top male sprinters when they reached a similar crossroads:

An athlete could not expect to win in top international competition without using anabolic steroids.

Steroids could not replace talent, or training, or a well-planned competitive program. They could not transform a plodder into a champion. But they had become an essential supplement at the world-class level, an indispensable ingredient within a complex recipe. (As Hermann Buhl, a top East German sports official, would later note, "We had that excellent coaching system, and [yet] it still was necessary at a certain period of history to add some pharmaceuticals.")

As I saw it, a coach had two options: He could face reality and plan an appropriate response, or he could bury his head in the sand while his athletes fell behind. The latter course was chosen by most of the Canadian coaching fraternity. While their stance protected them from public reproach, their athletes were left in a quandary. If they followed their coaches' credo, they effectively stunted their careers. If they didn't, they were forced to find other sources of information—like the black-market distributors who peddle their wares in gyms and health clubs. Left on their own, these athletes might not seek medical supervision. They would be exposed to greater risks of side effects and detection. And it would be scant consolation to them that their coaches remained above the fray.

Fairness was not a practical issue for us. In Canada, Angella had already left the competition far behind; it wouldn't change the placing were she to move farther in front. And on the international scene, our steroid program would make the playing field *more* level, not less.

Our sole concern, then, became one of safety: Would we risk Angella's health by using steroids? The more medical information I collected, the more my qualms were dispelled. I was heartened by the presentation of Dr. Doug Clement, the CTFA's respected medical director and an international anti-doping advocate, at the national coaches' meeting in Sherbrooke in July 1979. After one coach asked him to issue a statement about the health hazards of steroids, Clement replied that he couldn't do it. It simply wasn't true, he said: When regulated in small doses, there was no evidence that anabolic steroids had any significant side effects. Clement believed that they were no more dangerous than birth control pills (which steroids closely resembled), and substantially less dangerous than corticosteroids, anti-inflammatory drugs which are permitted by the IOC under limited and controlled circumstances.

Clement's opinion lay well within the mainstream of medical literature of the day. In a 1977 statement, the American College of Sports Medicine, while inveighing against the use of steroids and listing their potential side effects (including liver damage and reduced sperm production), went on to note that "these effects appear to be reversible when small doses of steroids are used for short periods of time." In *Anabolic Steroids and Sports*, James Wright, an exercise physiologist for the U.S. Army, observed that "dose and duration of use of oral anabolic and contraceptive steroids are the predominant factors influencing the development of hepatic lesions," including liver tumours.

Clement sought to end drug use in sport because he feared that an athlete who was prepared to use steroids would possess an unfair advantage over one who was not. He ruefully acknowledged, however, that his scruples were not universally shared within his profession. He said that many medical directors attended international anti-doping conferences as double agents—to obtain information for their athletes back home on the latest methods of skirting drug tests.

Angella and I resolved the issue that September. She had observed the changes in many of her top opponents, both in their bodies and their times. She made it clear that she had come too far to back off. If steroids were required to win, she wanted them.

In October 1979, as we prepared to resume training for the indoor season, Angella and I visited her personal physician, who had already been treating her for anæmia, a congenital condition which is especially common among black female athletes. While the doctor was uncertain about Dianabol's capacity to improve performance, he agreed to write a prescription for one five-milligram tablet a day. Like Clement, he foresaw no medical problems with a low dose.

(While I knew of two British female sprinters who were on 35 milligrams of Dianabol a day, my research suggested that much smaller doses could be effective—and could avert masculinizing side effects, including facial hair and a lowered voice register. As women produced relatively little male hormone to begin with, a given dose of steroids added more *proportionately* to a woman's system than it did to a man's.)

The doctor recommended that Angella take the Dianabol for three weeks at a time, with three weeks off between cycles—again agreeing with the literature I'd seen. The longer you maintained a steady-state dosage (the practice of certain American coaches), the greater the risk that the athlete's body might reduce, or even shut down, its own hormonal output. When the steroid dose was finally stopped, the body would enter a withdrawal state—a "crash" that might last for months, with repercussions for both health and performance. But if you constantly interrupted the drug's administration, so that each dose "shocked" the system, you would gain a maximum impact on performance with a minimal endocrine disturbance.

I knew there were steroid abusers out there, namely the body-builders, power lifters, throwers, and football players who took massive amounts of the drugs for extended periods of time. One power lifter known to us "stacked" (or combined) 150 milligrams of Dianabol, 200 milligrams of the particularly toxic Anadrol-50, and 100 milligrams of testosterone—a total of 450 milligrams a day, or (assuming a two-month off season) about *135,000* milligrams a year. At these megadoses, side effects might range from heart disease to diminished sex drive. As Clement and other experts had pointed out, however, the effects of *any* drug—from arsenic to aspirin—hinged on dosage and duration. In the early 1980s, the male sprinters in my group would take 3 percent or less of that lifter's daily dosage (with longer and more frequent interruptions), and the women in the group took much less than my men. According to Angella's first annual plan with steroids, she would take a *total* of about 700 milligrams for her indoor and outdoor seasons combined—less than the lifter would consume in two days.

From the start of her steroid regimen, Angella regularly checked her blood profile. The results were consistently normal. There were no evident side effects. But as predicted by her doctor, the steroid apparently raised Angella's hæmoglobin count and alleviated her anæmia.

For my part, I was relieved to have settled the issue. Given the pressures of the day, I believe I would choose the same course again. And I'd have plenty of company—and a venerable tradition on my side.

Steroids: A Brief History

The marriage between drugs and competition dates back millennia. Whenever winning has mattered, athletes have sought an edge over their rivals, never pausing to distinguish between the "natural" and the "artificial." Had the IAAF's banned list been in place in ancient Greece, many an Olympic champion might have lost his laurels for ingesting sheep's testicles—a prime source of testosterone. West Africans have used cola plants since antiquity to stave off fatigue in work and competition. Aztec athletes employed a cactus-based stimulant. And Norwegians tell stories of their Viking ancestors eating the fungus *Amanita muscaria*—a potent hallucinogen—to go berserk in battle, that bloodier cousin to sport.

The first documented modern case of doping surfaced in 1865, with Dutch swimmers using stimulants. By the late 19th century, according to Norwegian journalist Anne-Lise Hammer in her book *Doping Express*, European cyclists were widely drugging themselves with a variety of "miracle" products, from caffeine to ether-coated sugar cubes, to allay the pain and exhaustion endemic to their sport. French cyclists, in particular, were known to favour *Vin Mariani*, known as "wine for athletes," a compound of wine and coca leaf extract.

By the time of the first modern Olympics in 1896, a broad array of performance aids were in currency, from codeine to strychnine, a powerful stimulant in sub-lethal doses. Russian speed skaters were known to favour arsenic, while boxers of the day preferred brandy laced with strychnine or cocaine—a cocktail also endorsed by the American Thomas Hicks, an Olympic marathoner who won the gold in 1904. As noted by Michael Asken in *Dying to Win*, it took four physicians to revive Hicks after his triumph.

At the 1932 Olympics in Los Angeles, Japanese swimmers achieved an extraordinary success amid reports that they were inhaling oxygen in their locker room just before their events. Sprinters of the day experimented with nitroglycerine, in an effort to dilate the arteries of their hearts. But the modern age of doping dawned in 1935, when German scientists isolated testosterone. The Nazis injected the male sex hormone into their troops to make them more aggressive. They did the same for their athletes at the 1936 Olympics in Berlin, in an attempt to live up to their "super-race" billing. The German Olympians were also supplied with Pirvitan, a powerful amphetamine favoured by many European athletes to this day. (Jesse Owens notwithstanding, Germany went on to win the most medals at Berlin.)

The Germans' technology filtered into the Soviet Union after the Second World War, and came back to haunt the West in 1952, when the U.S.S.R. participated in its first Olympics in Helsinki and far surpassed expectations. At the 1956 Games in Melbourne, the Soviets won more medals than anyone else, and by then it was clear that their athletes were using testosterone. According to a contemporary account, however, the Russians were not alone in seeking an edge in Australia. "This craze for pills was most shocking at the recent Olympic Games," Neal Wilkinson wrote in *True* magazine in 1958. "In Olympic village, the athletes' rooms looked like small drug stores. Vials, bottles and pill boxes lined the shelves."

A pharmaceutical cold war was on, and with it the hunt for more advanced weapons. While straight testosterone helped people win, athletes were searching for something even better—a substance with greater anabolic (tissue-building) benefits, yet fewer side effects. In 1955, John Ziegler, the physician for the U.S. weightlifting team, developed a modified, synthetic testosterone molecule with enhanced tissue-building properties: the first man-made anabolic steroid. Its chemical name was methandrostenolone. Its trade name was Dianabol.

Developed by the Ciba Pharmaceutical Company of Basel, Switzerland, Dianabol was approved by the U.S. Food and Drug Administration to treat certain anæmias and skin diseases. (Anabolic steroids continue to be used to treat breast cancers, osteoporosis, severe anæmias, and testosterone deficiencies.) At the same time, the tablets launched an underground cult among athletes and body-builders. Those early initiates discovered, much as I would in 1973, that Dianabol could allay their fatigue, increase their muscularity, enhance their self-image and confidence, and—without a doubt, despite the medical establishment's denials into the 1980s—boost their performance.

Within the body, the steroid worked much like the hormone it was modelled after. It heightened ribonucleic acid (RNA) activity and spurred the synthesis of protein, the basic component of muscle, bone, and skin. It helped muscles to regenerate more quickly from the stress of training, in order to be stressed again. And for sprinters and other athletes in power events, the drug excited the motor neurons in their muscle fibres, resulting in faster muscle contractions—the foundation for higher speed and improved reaction times.

By the early 1960s, Dianabol had become indispensable to competitive weightlifters and the new wave of oversized pro football linemen in the U.S. According to one NFL player, coaches would place salad bowls of the tablets on their training tables. Players would scoop out pills by the handful and sprinkle them on their cereal—"the breakfast of champions," they called it. (Years after one player had estimated that three out of four NFL linemen were regular users, the league finally mounted a limited campaign against steroids, suspending a total of 17 players for either taking or distributing the drugs as of September 1990.)

The 1964 Olympics in Tokyo were the first Games to feature widespread steroid use by elite athletes from both sides of the Atlantic. It was most prevalent among throwers, whose world records surged an unlikely 12 percent during the decade. American runners resisted the wave at first, but they had joined the party by 1968—as I concluded, in retrospect, from their televised appearance at the Olympic trials at Lake Tahoe. I had seen the same athletes at their national championships only two months earlier, and the difference was profound and unmistakeable. They were both leaner and more muscular, with a smooth, rounded, almost waxy look.

Meanwhile, the use of stimulants among the cyclists had run rampant, and many were pushing their bodies past exhaustion and into trouble. In 1960, Knut Jensen of Denmark collapsed and died of heart failure during competition at the Rome Olympics, and anti-doping forces slowly began to stir. The IOC established its medical commission in 1967 and initiated testing for stimulants and narcotics at the following year's Olympics in Mexico City. But while the IOC banned a long list of drugs, including such peripheral substances as heroin and morphine, it ignored anabolic steroids. The athletes did not. By the 1972 Olympics in Munich, the insiders' consensus was that 80 percent of the top male competitors were using steroids, across the board of events—along with a number of women from East Germany, West Germany, the Soviet Union, and Britain.

After several media stories alleged widespread steroid use, the IAAF finally banned the drugs in 1975. By either mistake or design, however, the ban contained one huge loophole. The federation directed that steroids be treated exactly like stimulants—in other words, that athletes be tested for them only at competitions. In fact, the two types of drugs were categorically different, especially where runners were concerned. Amphetamines temporarily "fool" the nervous system into exceeding its normal capacity. To lend their instant advantage, stimulants must be in the athlete's body during an event. But steroids are *training* drugs, an investment for a future advantage. Users improve because they can train harder and faster—and superior training yields superior performances down the road. When a world-class athlete claims that he doesn't need steroids because he "works hard," he is stating a non sequitur. It is the steroids that *allow* him to work so hard—to increase his training capacity and withstand extreme physiological stress, thereby raising his performance level.

As I would find in 1982, the benefits of a steroid program carry over for months after an athlete goes "off the juice," in track jargon. Not only was it unnecessary for sprinters to stay on the drug in the last days before a meet, it would usually be a detriment to do so. Since steroids induce the body to retain more fluid, they might make sprinters too stiff to run their best.

In 1973, Professor Raymond Brooks of Britain, who developed the initial tests for anabolics, told the IAAF that any credible attack on steroid use would have to include random testing *outside* the competitions—to visit athletes unannounced during training and demand a urine test on the spot. (Robert Dugal, the Montreal lab director, expressed the same opinion in 1975, as did Doug Clement in an address at Canada's national coaches' meeting in 1979. But the CTFA would not institute random testing until after the scandal in Seoul in 1988—long after similar programs had been initiated in Britain, Sweden, and Norway.)

Meanwhile, the IOC and the IAAF, who were served by the same medical personnel, refused to admit that most of the best athletes were already using the drugs, and that Olympic qualifying standards—and the majority of world records—were steroid-dependent. The bureaucrats were boxed in. If they lowered the entry standards, they'd be jeopardizing the sport's image by conceding that the records had been set by steroid users. But if they left the standards intact, they would force competitors to violate the ban to survive. Without staying on steroids, no athlete could hope to surpass a world record which had been legally drug-aided. In more than a few events, people wouldn't even be able to make their nations' Olympic teams.

For anyone who continued to compete after 1975, the choice was clear: They could either break the rules or they could lose. Younger athletes who rose to prominence later on, like Angella Taylor and

Ben Johnson, faced the same alternatives. They had inherited a world in which steroids were *de rigueur*. As Angella would put it, "Nobody wants to be mediocre—nobody wants to be second best."

Meet testing made the steroid ban essentially unenforceable. Every steroid has a "clearance time," measured from the last dose, after which its metabolites can no longer be detected through a urine test. For oral Dianabol the accepted clearance time was 21 days. (To allow for a safety margin, I generally took my people off the drug at least 28 days before a tested meet.) To bridge the gap to race day, however, some athletes might switch to testosterone, for which there was no test until 1983; or take probenicid, which effectively masked steroid use and would be banned only in 1987; or add growth hormone, for which there is still no test. (Partly as a result of such manœuvres, only a tiny percentage of steroid users have ever been caught. Throughout two decades of acknowledged doping in East Germany, for example, only one G.D.R. athlete has failed a drug test at an international competition.)

The athletes soon came to perceive the steroid ban as a technicality, an arbitrary rule that no one followed. They were actively abetted by their coaches and national sports governing bodies—surreptitiously in the West, more openly within the Soviet bloc. According to Valentin Chumak, a Russian thrower of the '70s, the Soviets pre-tested all athletes before they entered the country's elite training centres. Officials wanted to be sure that these novices were not already using steroids—for purposes of uniformity in the state-controlled doping program, and so that the young athletes' potential could be accurately assessed. Hammer throwers, for example, were expected to improve by 10 metres after the centres put them on drugs. Anything less would be considered evidence of prior steroid use, and would be grounds for expulsion.

The full extent of the steroid ban fiasco became apparent at the 1976 Olympics, when the Soviets installed a fully equipped lab on their ship in Montreal's harbour for the duration of the Games. According to Chumak, urine samples were shuttled to the ship for secret testing before athletes began their events. This allowed them to continue taking their drugs to the last possible moment and still make sure they were clean. If they tested "dirty" at the ship, they would be pulled from the competition, thereby avoiding a scandal and suspension. This mattered most to the lifters and throwers, for whom raw strength counted far more than mobility, and who risked an endocrine crash—and a substantial drop-off in performance—if they discontinued their steroids too far in advance. The Soviets' advantage was even greater because they knew that the IOC's first-generation tests were more primitive than we'd assumed, and could not detect Dianabol beyond a clearance of five to seven days.

The Russians' gambit pointed up another problem with the steroid ban: the more rigorous the testing, the greater the handicap for athletes without access to state-of-the-art testing equipment. When our shot-put champion, Bishop Dolegiewicz, looked back at his disappointing performance in Montreal, it was with great bitterness. Canadian authorities had told Bishop that he needed at least a month off Dianabol to clear the test. They might as well have made him throw left-handed.

Floating laboratories were extreme measures, and rarely necessary. For the most part, dope testing remained sporadic until 1983. It was generally limited to the most important international competitions or to meets in cleaner-than-thou Britain, where officials often took pains to warn athletes about any potential risk, as we'd seen at our tri-meet in Gateshead. There were widespread rumours of cover-ups and trade-offs at international meets, which led athletes to shave their clearance times ever closer to the meets.

By 1979, when Angella was wrestling with her decision on steroids, it was becoming difficult to decipher the drug protocols without a degree in pharmacology. Dianabol, while still popular, was now being stacked with other, more event-specific steroids. In pursuits where body mass and strength mattered most (as in the throws and the heavyweight class of powerlifting), athletes were drifting toward more androgenic (or masculinizing) drugs, such as testosterone and Anadrol-50. In events where speed and mobility were paramount, and athletes wanted to add strength without bulking up or retaining too much water (as in the sprints), the trend was toward less androgenic steroids: Winstrol, Anavar, Primobolan. (To keep themselves slim, the latter group might use anabolics in conjunction with thyroxine, a thyroid supplement which speeds the metabolism.)

But while the game was getting more complicated, I had less and less doubt as to what we were up against. When I concluded that most of Angella's top competitors were already on steroids, I was not relying on idle gossip, nor on the vague sense that "everyone was doing it." My information came from trusted sources who were in a position to know.

Of the East Germans, whose women held every world sprint record of the day, there could be no doubt. In our women's 1979 dual meet with East Germany, a non-testing venue, our opponents had obviously come in loaded—at least 10 to 15 pounds heavier than at tested meets before and afterward. Several months later I filled in the blanks with the aid of a prominent West German coach who knew the G.D.R.'s Wolfgang Meier, Marita Koch's coach and husband. Meier had confirmed that East Germany's standard steroid protocol for women at that time ranged from 20 to 40 milligrams per day of Dianabol, with the individual's dose increased by 5 milligrams each year. In West Germany, according to my source, at least two top runners had followed the same protocol. I heard similar anecdotes about leading sprinters from other track powers, including the United States and Britain. I had no reason to doubt the stories—or to indict the athletes who were simply striving to stay abreast of their world-class rivals.

As Angella told an interviewer more than 10 years after she swallowed her first Dianabol tablet: "There's no athlete out there...who every day gets up and goes through a long moral dilemma—should I take this pill or should I not take this pill? You don't think about it.... First and foremost, what comes to mind is that this [pill] is going to help me become the best in the world."

Boycott

As my athletes progressed, coaching them became less mechanical and more intricate. There were so many components to their training—among them speed, strength, endurance, weight work, massage, and now, for Angella, steroids. Each one had its own optimal cycle, yet each was also a variable affected by all the others. Since the components overlapped (that is, we worked on several within a given period, or even on a single day), I had to be alert to their interactions. An unusually fast speed drill, for example, might prompt me to reduce or delete an athlete's weight work that day, since both activities taxed the neuromuscular system. At this level, coaching was never a static exercise. It was like working a jigsaw puzzle where the shapes of the pieces kept changing.

As my first world-class athlete, Angella Taylor bore the brunt of my trials and errors, particularly in how I played steroids against the other variables. In retrospect, I increased her workload beyond any boost in capacity she might have gotten from a five-milligram dose of Dianabol. (It would be several years before I understood that anabolics helped most by allowing us to raise the *intensity*, or pace, of our speed work, rather than the volume.) Ultimately, the overload would give rise to the injuries that stalled Angella's career. More immediately, it kept her from running to her full potential.

At the time, however, it was hard to gauge what I was doing right or wrong, because Angella was advancing so rapidly that *everything* seemed to work. She didn't crash when she went off the Dianabol, nor did she notably raise her game when she went back on. Her times kept improving, in linear fashion, throughout the year. That winter she set world indoor records in the 200 metres, the 300 yards, and the 300 metres. (Indoor records were somewhat less significant—since fewer world-class athletes compete indoors—than outdoor marks.) She dominated the Canadian track world so completely that she began to arouse the jealousy of the lesser lights around her.

In February 1980, at the national indoor championships, Angella came into the meet primed to break the world record of 23.19 for 200 metres. At the Metropolitan Toronto Track and Field Centre at York University, a new facility which had replaced the Pig Palace the year before, the third lane is fastest—the curve not too sharp, the banking just steep enough. We made it clear that Angella was going all out for the record, and that she expected to get lane three. Everyone knew that Angella was a second faster than her closest competition. As a Canadian running in a Canadian meet, she was requesting a courtesy routinely granted to premier runners in other nations.

Peter Manning, a coach who'd befriended our group, drew lane three for us in the semi-final, and Angella broke the world record in 23.15, despite some pain from a sore tendon. Manning would have done us the same favour for the final, but a meet official interceded and drew lane one for Angella—absolutely precluding a run at another record. I proposed that we scratch her from the final for health reasons—national championship or no—and both Angella and the team's doctor concurred. "I'll just let Molly win it," Angella said, referring to her clubmate, Molly Killingbeck.

"You can't scratch," a meet official protested. "People will think she's walking out because she didn't like the lane assignment."

"They might be right," I said.

Molly won the race.

Given the calibre of her indoor performances, Angella was now a legitimate contender for a medal in the 100 at the 1980 Olympics, to be held in Moscow that July. All told, nine of my athletes attained the Olympic standards in their events, including Desai, Ben, Tony, and Mark. They represented about half the Canadian Olympic sprint team. But at a June training camp in Los Angeles, we heard the dark rumours confirmed: that Canada would follow the United States' lead and boycott the Olympics in reaction to the Soviet invasion of Afghanistan.

Most of my sprinters weren't yet competitive at the world level, anyway. Ben's main concern was to gain carded status, which had been strangely denied him the previous fall. But Angella was devastated. She knew she was ready to compete against the best in the world. Later that summer, in Zurich, she beat four of the top five finishers in the Olympic final, including gold medallist Ludmila Kondratyeva of the Soviet Union and bronze medallist Ingrid Auerswald of East Germany. Angella had worked so hard to arrive at this point, and she knew too well the vagaries of her sport. Who could tell where she would be in 1984? "I've just got to win everything I can," she said to me, near tears.

Prime Minister Joe Clark, whose nine-month tenure happened to coincide with the pre-Olympic period, had knuckled under to American pressure to join the boycott. Canada wasn't the only nation to cave in. Guy Abrahams, a Panamanian sprinter who had attended USC and had trained with our group, had been assured that his home country would compete. At the eleventh hour, however, he received a call from the head of the Panamanian Olympic Committee. Panama would boycott after all, the official said; U.S. agents had bought up loans against his Panamanian company and had threatened to foreclose unless he fell into line.

Flag waving is fundamental to the Olympic experience. Whenever you attract a broad gathering of the world's press, you offer an instant platform for anyone whose voice is loud enough, from the swastika set at Berlin in 1936 to the Palestinians at Munich to all the

America boosters at Los Angeles in 1984. I tended to ignore the political hoopla, accepting it as the price of admission to the greatest
athletic show on earth. You cannot fund such a supreme competition without huge government subsidies—and, as on television, the
sponsors reserve the right to sell their wares.

But a boycott defeated everyone's purpose, even the politicians'.
It was a classic Carter miscalculation, a public relations stunt
whose chief attraction was that it would lose but a handful of
votes—namely those of the participants and their families. The
boycott's intended target, the Soviet Union, took the medals and
ran after scoring an unopposed propaganda coup, much as the
U.S. would four years later. The victims were not the commissars,
but the Free World's shackled athletes. One especially sad story
involved a world-ranked javelin thrower named Bruce Kennedy,
a Rhodesian national who attended school at Berkeley. In 1972,
he lost his Olympic chance when Rhodesia, with its pariah white-
minority regime, was expelled from the Games. In 1976, the year
that more than two dozen other African nations boycotted the
Montreal Olympics over a New Zealand rugby team's tour of
South Africa, Rhodesia was so paralysed by internal conflict that
it could not organize a team. Still a world-class athlete, Kennedy
figured he would solve his geopolitical problems by obtaining U.S.
citizenship. He made the U.S. team in 1980, only to be done in by
Carter even as his native country (now Zimbabwe) was readmitted
to the Olympics and allowed to take part in the Moscow Games.

As a pallid substitute for the Olympics, the U.S. sponsored a
"Freedom Games" meet for its allies in Philadelphia that summer.
Angella won the 200 against the top American and Western Euro-
pean sprinters, did the same at a similar meet in Stuttgart, and went
on to win at least one sprint in every Grand Prix meet except for
Zurich, where she finished second in the 100 to world-record holder
Marlies Göhr. At the end of the season, *Track & Field News* ranked
her fifth in the world in the 100 metres.

Desai placed third in the 100 at both Philadelphia and Stuttgart.
Ben, meanwhile, finished fifth at Stuttgart after placing second to

Desai at the Canadian nationals in a personal best of 10.36; at the age of 18, he was beginning to tap his vast talent.

Less Is More

By the fall of 1980, I had 11 carded athletes (including Ben, for the first time)—about one-third of my group. In spite of my success, I was still unpaid as a coach and would stay that way a while longer, living on a shoestring.

That fall, Sport Ontario (the province's counterpart to Sport Canada) approved funding for a two-year pilot project to foster high performance in the sprints. The project's staff, to be appointed by the Ontario Track and Field Association, would consist of an "apprentice coach," at a salary of $20,000 a year, and a supervising "master coach," who would receive a $4,000 annual stipend for his limited part-time work. Gerard Mach was the manifest choice for the master coaching position, and my record made me the obvious candidate for the apprenticeship. But neighbouring clubs had long resented the Optimists' dominance, and I was distinctly *persona non grata* in provincial track circles. The job went to Peter Green, an Ottawan who had never placed a sprinter on the national team. And the master's stipend, rather than going to Gerard, who also lived in Ottawa and was ideally placed to oversee Green's work, went instead to Rolf Lund, the president of the OTFA and a member of the CTFA's board of directors, who lived 100 miles away in Kingston.

(Two years later, after Sport Ontario cancelled the project, Lund managed to get funding for a second two-year master coaching stint in the pole vault, and finally, a third for the high jump. Each time Lund was named master coach; in the end, after six years of non-production, the provincial coaching project was cancelled.)

After working without a salary for nearly three years, I had to sell my Aston Martin to repay $17,000 in credit card debts. But my financial strain was relieved on April 1, 1981, when the National Sprint Centre officially opened for business at York University, and I was installed as coach. The federal mandate behind the centre system was to promote world-class performance with a minimal capital investment. My athletes, who would form the core of the new program, would work out at York as before, and the Optimists would continue to support our training camps, tours, and equipment. The centre's initial budget totalled only $54,000— including $25,000 for my salary—with Sport Canada and Sport Ontario each contributing half. The funds would be administered by the CTFA. The OTFA, which had lobbied against the centre, was frozen out. It was a power play by Sport Canada, which knew that funding for future centres in other sports, such as swimming and gymnastics, would hinge on the sprinters' performances. Sport Canada couldn't afford a patronage appointment; this pilot project had to work.

My top athletes were beginning to attract attention on the world scene. Ben and Tony, in particular, were moving steadily ahead. If there was a turning point in Ben's career, a single race which predicted his future, it came in August 1981, at the World Cup trials in Venezuela. Only 19 years old, Ben ran second in 10.25, the fastest 100-metre time yet within my group and a Canadian junior record. Though still about two-tenths of a second behind the world's best senior sprinters of the day, Ben's race showed how far our world had turned in 10 years; it was roughly equivalent to a hand-timed

10-flat, Valery Borzov's world-best time in 1971. Later that summer, Ben leaped over Desai and Tony to become the first Canadian to reach the finals in all three of Europe's most competitive meets: Zurich, Berlin, and Cologne. The Zurich *Weltklasse* final was considered the most exclusive in the sport, including the Olympics. (Zurich was tougher because the Americans could flood the meet, while the Olympics limited them to three entries. In 1984, it would require a 10.32 to make the Olympic final in the 100 metres—and a 10.16 to make the final at Zurich.)

While Ben didn't place in any of these meets, he opened eyes with his explosive starts, a product of his unique, leaping style, his tautly tuned nervous system, and his growing strength. At Zurich he ripped out of the blocks and led the field through 50 metres— he must have been running at an electronic 10-flat pace—before falling back, his energy burned, to finish last in 10.40. (I encouraged Ben to go all out from a race's start; I believed that sprinters had a finite "envelope" of energy to draw from on any given day, and that their final time would be the same whether they drew from it early or drew from it late.) Mel Lattany, the American who won the race in 10.09, was astounded: "How did you learn to start like that?" With his characteristic shy confidence, Ben replied, "Just natural, mon."

Like the rest of my top male sprinters, Ben wasn't yet strong enough to run to the finish with the likes of Lattany. But unlike Desai, Tony, or Mark, Ben never worried about the competition and seldom froze under pressure. He stayed calm, running as fast as he could for as long as he could. I discovered that Ben, like Angella, was that rare track phenomenon: a big-money player, one who came through when the stakes were high. It was relatively easy to add speed endurance to a maturing sprinter; it was far harder to add poise. That European summer took Ben's measure, and he met every test.

It was in 1978, from a Clemson athlete named Steve Davis, that I first got wind of the talented schoolboy who was already building his legend. "There's a guy named Carl Lewis," said Davis, who came from the same New Jersey town. "He's 16 years old and jumped 26 feet." I didn't believe it at first, since such a leap would have landed a spot in the 1976 Olympic finals. But I subsequently found that Davis had scarcely been exaggerating; the Willingboro High School student he'd touted had indeed jumped 25 feet, 9 inches that summer.

As late as 1979, Carl Lewis remained an outstanding high school long jumper who ran the 100 metres in the 10.50s—solid, but nothing remarkable. When I first met Carl in July of that year, at the Pan Ams in Puerto Rico, he had reached his adult height of six-two, but he still had the skinny body of an adolescent.

Just one year later, I watched amazed as Lewis burst upon the international scene at a meet in the Netherlands where he finished a fast-closing second to Stan Floyd, then the world's top-ranked sprinter. Since enrolling at the University of Houston in the fall of 1979, Lewis had pared his personal best to 10.21 and looked like he'd put on 25 pounds of muscle. In August 1980, at the Pan Am juniors in Sudbury, Ontario, Carl and Ben hooked up for the first time; Carl won the race in 10.43, while Ben finished sixth in 10.88. By 1981, Lewis was running 10-flat, and an international superstar was born. At the end of that season, he was ranked first in the 100 by *Track & Field News*, the first of five consecutive years he would hold the most coveted and lucrative title in sport: The World's Fastest Human.

The Sprint Centre budget allowed me to hire a physiotherapist, someone who could tend to my athletes' injuries and take on most of the massage. Early that summer, shortly before our national championships, I interviewed my first applicant: Mike Dincu, a 32-year-old fire plug of a man who radiated frightening enthusiasm. Super Mike, as he liked to be called, was a recent Romanian defector who'd served that nation's top soccer team. (The best physios were all defectors from the ultra-organized sports systems of Eastern Europe. In North America, people with Mike's training and expertise simply didn't exist.)

Super Mike didn't have a work uniform at the time, so he gave me a trial massage while dressed in a T-shirt, jockey shorts, and sandals. I could tell he was good straight away and hired him on the spot. A tireless worker, Super Mike never counted the hours he put in, and was even willing to tackle the throwers' huge muscles. He was also a character of the first order. After living in a rigidly structured and rationed society, Super Mike suddenly found he could say—and eat—anything he liked, and proceeded to do so with a vengeance. When he saw a 200-pound woman on the street, he looked her in the eye and said: "Tell me, what you eat to get so fat?" His own dinners were multi-course orgies in which he'd shovel down the food, barely pausing to breathe.

The 1981 nationals went well, with Angella and Desai sweeping the individual sprints, and then we were off to Venezuela for the World Cup trials. The trip was interminable; the U.S. air controllers' strike caused a four-hour delay in Toronto and a seven-hour layover in Miami before we could take off for Caracas. I had just settled into my seat on the latter flight when a woman ran past me through the aisle, screaming, "They've caught a Russian spy! They've caught a Russian spy!" As Miami police and airport security people boarded the plane, I had a sinking feeling. Then a stewardess told me what was going on: Super Mike had claimed he had a bomb in his bag. At first I couldn't believe he could get into this much trouble—the man could barely speak English. But Super Mike was fluent in Spanish, and he'd decided to charm the Hispanic stewardess with a little joke—that he had Atomic *Balm*, a heat rub, in his suitcase.

We straightened that much out (and were fortunate to save our physio from criminal charges), but the captain was not amused. "Get him and his bags out of here," he commanded. "This plane isn't leaving with him." Super Mike was dispatched back to Toronto. Now I would have to do all the massages in Venezuela; by the end of the meet, I would be sorer than my runners.

But Super Mike was nothing if not persistent. Anxious to redeem himself, he arranged for another plane ticket from the CTFA and flew out to Caracas. There was only one problem: He had no idea where to go from there. "World Cup, World Cup!" he would say to anyone he could buttonhole. Someone found a publicity brochure which advertised the trials in the coastal city of Cumaná, about 200 miles east. Super Mike caught another plane, but when he landed in Cumaná—"World Cup, World Cup!"—he discovered that the meet had been moved to Ciudad Bolívar, 150 miles to the south. By the time Super Mike finally found us, the trials were almost over. The punch line came when the CTFA billed me for $1,100 for my physio's extra flight.

At an IAAF coaching symposium in Venice that season, I crossed paths with the world's pre-eminent women's sprint coach: Horst Hille of the Motor City Jena Club in East Germany. Hille's English was almost as limited as my German, and he was rather guarded at the start, deferring to the smoother Edwin Tepper, the G.D.R.'s head women's coach. But Hille was the man who had developed such champions as Renate Stecher, Marlies Göhr, and Bärbel Wöckel, the 1976 and 1980 Olympic gold medallist in the 200 metres. My persistent questioning wore him down, and one afternoon he haltingly outlined his program.

To begin with, Hille's resources went far beyond anything I had known in North America, or in Western Europe for that matter, or even in Gerard's heyday in Poland. "I put in my plan and whatever I want, that's it," Hille told me. "There's no discussion." Motor City Jena had exclusive call on two apartment buildings, a hotel, a fleet of buses and cars, and its own DC-9 to fly to training camps anywhere in the world. To serve a group of 30 sprinters, Jena employed a support staff of 21 doctors, sports scientists, technicians, physiotherapists, and masseurs; for my own slightly larger group, I had Mike Dincu. Where my top runners subsisted on starvation-level carding subsidies (if they were lucky), Hille could give a promising 17-year-old her own apartment and car, in addition to a decent salary. A top sprinter might make twice as much as the G.D.R.'s most successful industrial manager; a superstar like Marlies Göhr earned as much as the nation's president.

To recruit, Hille skimmed the cream of a rigorously organized national program for female sprinters. By the time they got to Hille, these young women were fully developed athletes; to be accepted in the Jena club, a girl had to run at least 11.50 in the 100 metres, a European junior championship level. By contrast, I was working with girls who came in at 12.90 or 13-flat.

(The G.D.R.'s program for males was entirely separate and, according to Tepper, in tremendous disarray, with no uniformity in training and deficient preparation at the lower levels. As a result, the East German men were not nearly as successful internationally—a failing which persisted even after Tepper took charge of them in 1982.)

In direct opposition to North American conventions, Jena's sprinters began their training at top speed and short distances, then stretched out as the season progressed. Hille understood that power athletes responded better to this pattern, since it played to their strengths. This philosophy was universal among East German coaches. Their swimmers, for example, used a water treadmill that was dialled into a world-record pace from early in the season. To maintain their position against the resistance, the swimmers had to sustain the same gruelling pace. At first they might go only 30 metres before falling back. But as they built their fitness, they would last longer and longer—until, at peak, they could go at a record pace from start to finish.

I had long before sensed that maximum velocity was the primary factor in sprinting, and that speed endurance must be built in at the desired pace, but the East Germans had applied the theory systematically, and with the highest technology. When Marita Koch was training to break the 400-metre world record, she would run on a track ringed by 80 computer-controlled timing lights, set five metres apart to flash at the desired race pace. All she had to do was to follow the lights.

Hille's greatest contribution to my own coaching methods lay in his taper schedule—his system for reducing his sprinters' training volume before a big meet. To guard against miscommunication, I sketched a blank schedule on a sheet of paper. I worked backwards;

I wrote "Olympic Games" at the bottom of the sheet, then worked up from there by jotting the numbers 1 through 10, with each number representing one more day before the event.

My own taper schedule was already extreme among North Americans. To keep my sprinters fresh, I generally planned my last full-scale speed work-out for five days before a competition, as compared to the three-day taper used by most of my peers. I believed it was that work-out—in its timing, volume, and intensity—which had the single greatest impact on a sprinter's subsequent performance, and I wanted to see how Hille's plan compared.

Hille methodically filled in the blanks, in the spirit of coaching fraternity—a spirit probably warmed by the fact that I'd given him a bottle of top-shelf Canadian whisky and 20 packs of cigarettes. I wondered at first if he had misunderstood. But there was no mistake—only my silent amazement at the numbers he'd placed on the page. At Motor City Jena, sprinters ran their last full-speed work-outs *10* days before their meets—an unheard-of gap in the West.

There were more surprises. During that last maximum work-out, Hille's women sprinters performed about as much speed work as mine did, but at an even higher intensity—in some cases at world-record paces. Hille's athletes would run four 30-metre starts, with seven-minute rests between them. They then took a 15-minute break, followed by an 80-metre sprint; then a 20-minute break and a 100-metre sprint; then a 25-minute break and a 120-metre sprint; finally, a 35-minute break and a 150-metre sprint. These were extraordinary rest periods—my own sprinters had never paused longer than 15 minutes between speed runs at those distances, and most coaches allowed for rests of five minutes or less.

These extended recoveries, along with the East Germans' incomparable massage, physiotherapy, and other support, allowed their sprinters to go at their absolute maximum on that 10th day before the meet. The work was of such high quality that a sprinter's central nervous system—first drained by the intense speed, then recharged by the ten-day taper period—would rebound like a pogo stick on the day of the competition. (To use the technical term, the sprinter would "super-compensate" to an even higher peak than at the last maximum work-out.) In between—usually on the eighth, sixth, fourth, and second days preceding the meet—Hille's sprinters would perform a single speed drill, either 80 or 120 metres, at 95 percent of maximum intensity. In these work-outs they were simply keeping their muscles tuned, without deepening fatigue.

Through exhaustive research (and, undoubtedly, much trial and error), the East Germans had found the keys to the kingdom of international track: the optimal balance of work and rest to ensure that their athletes would perform at their absolute best when it counted most.

Where Percy Duncan had taught me how to run and Gerard Mach how to plan, Horst Hille showed me how to carry my "less is more" philosophy to its logical—and winning—conclusion. By 1982, I had incorporated his taper schedule into my training program. I could never match the G.D.R. coaches in resources or support staff. Nor, lacking a formal feeder network, could I expect to produce world-record holders by the bunches. But my training regimen—a synthesis of my own methods and the innovations I had gleaned from the masters of my craft—had reached a level unprecedented in Canada. With this applied to the right sprinter, I began to believe that there might be no limit to how far we could go.

Crossroads

Angella's outdoor season was stunted by a June injury that was clearly my fault. Our over-training had left her muscles too highly toned going into her first outdoor meet, in Fürth, West Germany—a condition that may have been aggravated by her taking steroids through the untested competition. (She set a new Canadian record for the 100 at that meet in 11.12.) Four days later Angella strained her hamstring in Bratislava. She was injured again while winning the World Cup trials, but recovered well enough to run fourth in both the 100 and 200 at the World Cup in Rome.

That World Cup was most memorable for the Great Deca-Durabolin Scare. Deca was an oil-based, injectable steroid which was prized for its effectiveness. (To this day, it remains the body-builder's enhancement of choice.) The drug was especially popular in East Germany, which reportedly consumed more than half of the world's production. People liked Deca so much that they tended to push their luck with its clearance time, which was significantly longer than that of oral steroids like Dianabol or water-based injectables like Winstrol-V. But only a few of the savviest steroid veterans suspected *how* much longer—that the latest testing procedures could detect Deca anywhere from 6 to 13 months after the last dose. The panic broke when Ben Plucknett, the world-record holder in the discus, tested positive for Deca-Durabolin at the Pacific Conference Games in New Zealand and was suspended in June, just two months before the World Cup. Numerous athletes pulled out of the meet, many more than usual, including several prominent Americans for whom last-minute replacements were found. It was the first time that an advance in drug testing disrupted a competition, but it would not be the last.

Up to this point, none of my men had reached the level where steroids were a prerequisite for success. But now Desai, Ben, and Tony were approaching Angella's crossroads of two years before. They had become good enough to compete at the world level, yet their counterparts from other countries were starting to pull away from them.

At Fürth I was watching my runners practise when Brian Old-field, the top American shot-putter, confronted me. "When are you going to start getting serious?" he demanded. "When are you going to tell your guys the facts of life?" I asked him how he could tell they weren't already using steroids. He replied that the muscle density just wasn't there. "Your guys will never be able to compete against the Americans—their careers will be over," he persisted.

With that, Oldfield proceeded to tell me about an eminent U.S. sprint coach who had become an expert on steroids after joining a testosterone study with collegiate athletes, and about a woman who'd been a mediocre performer in the States before her coach put her on 35 milligrams of Dianabol, whereupon she became world-ranked. (The latter story was no surprise to me, since I'd been told of a second woman athlete with the same coach who had made similar strides with Dianabol.)

Like Oldfield, I'd seen visible and dramatic changes of late in American and European athletes, particularly in the junior ranks. In 1977, Desai was beating the people in his age group. But a year later, though he had continued to make good progress, a number of athletes had leapfrogged over him to world-ranked positions. I'd seen first-hand the abrupt improvements made by several of those runners, along with their new beach-movie physiques. I didn't need to see a dripping needle to grasp what was going on.

Back home, meanwhile, I had the example of John Smith, the American 400-metre runner who had moved in the fall of 1980 to Toronto, where he'd trained with me for several months. Smith told me he had begun taking 25 milligrams of Dianabol per day in 1970 while at UCLA, and in one year had improved from 47-flat to 45-flat. It seemed clear that such performance leaps couldn't be ascribed to training alone, no matter how "hard" people worked.

While the track federations had stiffened their public anti-drug stance and (sporadically) their testing and enforcement, they continued to wink at the steroid epidemic. A few months after Ben Plucknett tested positive and was banned, The Athletics Congress (the Americans' equivalent of the CTFA) presented him with its award for the year's outstanding performance.

I had skirted the issue in 1979 and 1980 by enrolling Desai and the others at Clemson University, where I assumed that steroids would be designed into their training. I was at least half-right; according to my athletes, they were each given a bottle of Dianabol tablets and told to take one per day, with no discussion of their going on and off the drug at set intervals—what we would come to refer to as "cycling." There were conflicting stories as to whether any of them had taken the drug—but even if they had, they hadn't used enough to create any noticeable effect. In any case, Clemson was history. As with Angella, it would be up to me to broach the subject.

While Desai and Tony knew the score from their college days, Ben had been left to draw his own conclusions from what he saw on the circuit. In September 1981, three months before Ben's 20th birthday, we met privately for a long discussion about his training for the coming year, which would culminate in the Commonwealth Games. Ben had never liked our 300-metre special endurance runs in practice—he felt they sapped his strength—and proposed limiting his longest drills to 200 metres. I took his request seriously, since Ben usually deferred to me, and agreed to the revision for that fall.

Then our conversation turned to steroids. It was immediately apparent that Ben understood how widespread they were, that he saw who was improving and why. I told him what I knew. I estimated that steroids represented at least one percent of performance—or one metre in the 100—at the elite level. Though the decision to take the drugs was Ben's, he had little choice if he agreed with my conclusions. He could either set up his starting blocks on the same line as his international competition, or he could start a metre behind.

Ben agreed that I should arrange a meeting with the doctor, who told him the same story he'd related to Angella in 1979—that Dianabol's side effects were essentially nil at the doses under discussion. A few days later Ben called me to say he had decided: He wanted to use steroids.

After Desai and Tony came independently to the same decision, the three men initially went on Angella's protocol of the year before: five milligrams of Dianabol per day, to be taken in three-week, on-and-off cycles. (Later that season, the men would alternate five milligrams one day and 10 milligrams the next.) As the Canadian manufacturer of Dianabol had voluntarily withdrawn it from the market (though it continued to be approved for use by prescription), I purchased several 100-tablet bottles at $25 apiece from Bishop Dolegiewicz, the Canadian champion shot-putter, and gave one bottle to each of the men. I made it clear that no pills were to be taken within 28 days of a meet and that they should visit their own physicians for regular blood tests.

Without fanfare or moralizing, our drug program was in place.

A few years later, after we had achieved prominence on the world scene, rival coaches in Canada would deride me as "Charlie the Chemist" and suggest that my success rested on my group's use of steroids. They ignored the fact that my runners ruled the Canadian track scene *before* our men's drug program began, just as Angella had won the nationals before she went on Dianabol. In both 1980 and 1981, I coached seven of eight finalists in the men's 100 metres at the Canadian nationals. By the end of the 1981 season, Ben had improved to 10.25, Desai to 10.26, and Tony to 10.31, while their closest Canadian competitors in the 100 were mired in the 10.70s and 10.80s. Among them, my three top male sprinters had broken a string of Canadian records, both indoors and outdoors, before they had taken drugs.

In addition, I had reason to suspect that my athletes were not the first Canadian sprinters to use banned substances. Marv Nash, a Montreal-based sprinter who'd been a member of the Canadian relay team which competed at the Pan American Games in Mexico City in 1975, told me that two other Canadian runners were so concerned about an impending drug test there that they asked Marv to fill their bottles with his urine. As the testing room was unguarded, he co-operated.

Of the 24 carded athletes I coached, 10 eventually used drugs under my direction, but the remaining 14 did not. If an athlete resisted the idea of steroids—as did Charmaine Crooks, who won the 400 metres in the national championships of 1979 and 1980—I never pressed. In one case, that of the 18-year-old Tony Issajenko (who would marry Angella in 1985), I dissuaded a runner from going on Dianabol for fear that it might stunt his growth. I always regarded the decision to use drugs as an individual choice, rather than a team policy.

At the same time, I knew that steroids were an essential part of a world-class program. We were prepared to fulfill Sport Canada's mandate: to develop sprinters who could compete at the highest level. No one familiar with international track and field could have imagined that we would get there drug-free.

Commonwealth Champs

We were all maturing, athletes and coach together. To this point, I had played the autocrat with my sprinters, demanding that they show up on time and do precisely what I wanted at practice. I generally got my way, but at the expense of resentment from my more independent athletes, such as Desai. When we resumed training in the fall of 1981, I decided to change. I stopped taking attendance and no longer rode herd over people in practice; I became less of a parent and more of a friend. In the long run, no amount of hectoring can substitute for self-discipline. No coach can push a runner to the top.

I rented a three-bedroom apartment within walking distance of the track, and the place became a crash pad for sprinters coming to us from out of town. Some would stay for a day or two; others, like Mike Sokolowski and Andrew Mowatt, for months at a time. Even after they were carded, many of my athletes did not have enough money to make it on their own. If they trained and went to school, there was no time for a paying job. The Sport Canada stipends—then a uniform $450 a month—could cover their rent, or it could buy food and other essentials, but not both. When I learned that two of my carded sprinters, Cheryl Thibedeau and

Rosey Edeh, were dining on Fruit Loops, I began stocking their kitchen with groceries. And I listened patiently to countless stories of homesickness and failed love affairs. My interest was real, but it was also part of my job. When athletes have problems and no one to turn to, their training quickly suffers.

At the track I did my best to foster communication. My top sprinters had mastered the fundamentals; now they required more customized training. A mass prescription would never work. To the extent that they were conscious of their bodies, the athletes themselves were the best judges of what helped them most—and when they'd done enough. Since my top sprinters were now outrunning my own personal bests, and I could no longer *feel* what they were going through, this feedback was my most reliable gauge. The students had surpassed the teacher.

This was especially true for Ben, who had an almost mystical self-awareness on the track. More than any of my other sprinters, he could sense precisely how fast he was going and could alter his pace to order. If I told him to run a 150-metre drill two-tenths of a second slower than his last one, an almost imperceptible difference, he modulated with ease. When I offered a technical suggestion—to lift his heels higher as they came up underneath him, for example—he understood and complied without missing a beat.

My new, more participatory approach toward training paid immediate dividends with Ben. He became a noticeably fresher runner after I deleted the 300-metre runs from his program, as he'd requested, and at no cost to his stamina. With Angella, who would compulsively override her internal warning signals, I needed to watch more closely for signs of fatigue. (Later on I tore up Angella's written work-out schedules. I knew that she would otherwise do every last drill at every single practice, even if she was exhausted. Instead I would assign her one task at a time. When I saw that she was tiring, I ended the work-out.)

While I would continue to tinker in seasons to come, especially with our drug protocol, the training program that would carry us to Seoul was essentially in place by the spring of 1982. I adapted Hille's taper schedule and trimmed our pre-competition speed work. By the time we concluded a sprint dual meet with the United States in Colorado Springs in mid-July, the first returns were in: We had reached the next level. Exploiting the high altitude, Angella won the 200 in 22.25, a Canadian record, and the 100 in 11.03, a Commonwealth record and the second-fastest performance in the world that year. (The Europeans had yet to weigh in with their major meets.) Tony also won both sprints, in 10.19 (just two hundredths off Jerome's Canadian record) and 20.22, which placed him third on the world list for the 200 metres. Our men's and women's 4x100 relay teams won as well, and both broke Canadian records. It was a coup for the Optimists and for me in particular; six of the eight relay runners were mine.

The biggest surprise was Ben's performance in a second running of the 200 metres, an event he entered as a "rabbit," to provide a fast early pace for Desai. Ben would run the 200 less and less frequently as his career evolved. Aside from his aversion to longer distances, he found the event superfluous, since the 100 metres alone bestowed the title of world's fastest human. Moreover, the meet promoters would pay no more to an athlete for running in an extra event. Had Ben regularly entered both sprints, the cumulative fatigue would have hurt his 100-metre times by season's end.

On this afternoon, however, Ben hinted that he would have excelled in the 200 had he worked at it. To Desai's chagrin, Ben led from the start and won the race in a wind-aided 20.37. Even adding a tenth or two for the wind, he'd far outstripped his previous personal best of 21.33. The rabbit had forgotten to stop.

In June, a month before the meet in Colorado Springs, we'd embarked on an overseas tour to Yugoslavia and Italy. I was concerned about drug testing in these dual-meet competitions. To keep our athletes peaking through the summer, our optimal steroid protocol would require them to continue taking the drug up to 21 days before the meet in Yugoslavia, or seven days shy of our normal safety margin. At an April meeting with Don Fletcher, director general of the CTFA, I asked him to find out if there would be testing at either meet. He phoned me two weeks later and said there would be none.

In Yugoslavia, the major excitement came after the meet, when local police visited our hotel in search of two Canadian team officials. After a few drinks too many at a reception earlier that evening, the two had liberated a portrait of Marshal Tito from the town hall. The police retrieved the picture and let the officials off with a warning.

At the second meet, in Venice, I got a taste of international gamesmanship. In Europe, track is a matter of national pride. Countries are prepared to defend their position by tactics fair or foul, and none more so than Italy. The Italians moved the women's meet—where Canada was sure to win—to a remote rural track. To further limit press coverage, they slotted the women's events on the night of the World Cup soccer finals. And to guarantee that there would be no noteworthy performances, all sprints were run into a headwind.

In the men's competition, a tight match on paper, we were felled by the home officials. In the walking event, the Italian athletes were breaking into a run on the far side of the track. When a Canadian did the same and got the lead, he was promptly disqualified. But the biggest insult came during the 4x100 relays, which our men figured to win easily. We were well ahead when anchor Sterling Hinds fumbled the baton on the pass and was run down by the Italian anchor. I wondered what had happened, since our passes were normally reliable. Then I asked Sterling to hand me the baton— and discovered that it was only nine inches long, about 60 percent of regulation length! Sterling simply hadn't been able to get a firm grip on it. That was a trick I'd never seen before—the Italians had short-sticked us.

The CTFA had begun meet testing in 1981 (three years before The Athletics Congress in the States), and we knew it would test the 1982 national championships in Ottawa in late July. After three years of Optimist domination, rival Canadian coaches hoped that our performances at sea level would fall short of our superlative times at Colorado Springs. They knew that we'd discontinued our steroids for the season two months before, and they assumed we would be off form. They didn't understand that steroids were training drugs; they mistakenly believed that our sprinters could do their best only during the periods that they were taking their pills.

I was beginning to learn, however, that our athletes could go drug-free far longer than anticipated without a crash—in part because of our low-dose protocol, in part because we maintained our tempo running throughout the season, which kept people lean and fit. Angella won the 100 in Ottawa in 11.07, the fastest time ever run on Canadian soil—faster than the winning time in the 1976 Olympics or the 1979 World Cup. She went on to take the 200 by more than a second, while Tony and Desai swept the men's sprints.

As my top sprinters began to run in more major meets, and therefore needed to peak over longer periods, I began looking for a drug that might be used through the Grand Prix series in Europe. (None of the Grand Prix meets was tested at the time.) I sought something milder than Dianabol—a steroid that wouldn't make our sprinters stiff in Europe, yet would keep them at their peak into the Commonwealth Games in Australia that October, our most important competition of the year. At the nationals I asked Bishop Dolegiewicz for advice, and he suggested oral stanozolol, known as Winstrol—it caused less fluid retention than other steroids, he said. He sold me a supply of two-milligram tablets, and advised that we use six milligrams as a standard daily dose. I distributed a two-weeks' supply to Angella, Desai, Ben, and Tony. Seven days into the protocol, after our first meet on the circuit in Berne, all four reported severe stiffness in their legs and stopped taking the drug. I could only hope that the Dianabol we'd administered in May would be sufficient for the remainder of the season.

The first good sign came in Europe, where Angella won six Grand Prix races, including Zurich for the first time. We met even tougher competition in September, at the Eight Nations Meet in Tokyo, which featured such powers as the United States, the Soviet Union, and East and West Germany. Angella led off by shocking the G.D.R.'s undefeated and heavily favoured Bärbel Wöckel in the 200 and then, though exhausted, running second to top-ranked Marlies Göhr in the 100. In an almost equally wild upset, Desai defeated Olaf Prenzler, the G.D.R.'s European champion, in the 200. After the two Canadians were voted the meet's outstanding athletes, our group was no longer the track world's best-kept secret.

One month later, we certified our new status at the Commonwealth Games in Brisbane, the quadrennial get-together of Britain and her former colonies. As expected, my athletes stacked the Canadian sprint team. It was less expected, however, that they would drub the best of Britain, Australia, and Jamaica.

As it turned out, everyone rose to the occasion. Angella broke the Commonwealth record in the 100 in 11-flat, defeating NCAA champion Merlene Ottey, then took a bronze in the 200. She also won a silver on our 4x100 women's relay team, and—as a last-minute replacement and anchor—a gold in the 4x400. Ben, recovered from a knee problem, ran a surprising second in the men's 100 with a wind-aided 10.05, a mere three hundredths behind Allan Wells, the Olympic champion. Wells just caught him at the tape; had Ben held form for another two metres, he would have won. (Tony and Desai, who ran in adjacent lanes, lost all chance in the race when they bumped arms at the 60-metre mark. At that they did better than former Olympic champions Hasely Crawford and Don Quarrie, who couldn't make the final.)

An all-Optimist 4x100 men's relay team, consisting of Ben, Desai, Tony, and Mark, took the silver, but the *coup de grâce* came in the men's 110-metre hurdles. Mark, who was ranked only fifth in the field going in, applied heat rub to his legs shortly before his race. But he put on too much and within seconds was in agony. He tried to remove the incendiary ointment, but his hairy legs stymied him. Mark began buzzing around the warm-up track like a hot-foot victim, then hopped into a shower—the worst thing he could have done, since it only opened his pores to the stuff. By the time he lined up for the event, he was jumping out of his skin. As I watched him move to a large and early lead, it became apparent that something wonderful was happening. The heat rub had apparently burned off any pre-race anxiety. Mark crossed the line in 13.37: a gold medal, a new Commonwealth record, three hundredths faster than the winning time at the 1980 Olympics, and more than four tenths better than Mark's previous personal best.

The Commonwealth Games represented our first great international triumph. My athletes came away with 13 medals, but I was almost too weary to enjoy it. The Sport Medicine Council of Canada had flown out a flock of physiotherapists, yet not a single masseur. The physios had no idea how to rub an athlete properly; their attempts were anæmic at best.

Gerard Mach was spoiling for a fight. "What are you going to do for massage?" he demanded at a staff meeting.

"We've got eight tons of equipment here," one of the physios said.

"You can take your machines and throw them in the ocean!" Gerard shouted. "How are you going to help the athletes prepare— wait until they're injured and then put them in a splint?"

The physios' answer was to bring in a table, a pile of towels, and a jug of oil—and leave the job to me. Every day I'd come in from the track at 5:30 P.M., wolf down my dinner, and massage the athletes till 1:00 A.M.—not only my own group, but anyone who needed it.

My low-budget band of Optimists had come far. We were now beyond question the top sprint group in the Commonwealth, and respected contenders at any international meet we entered. In my first full year as a paid coach, my runners had recorded 89 personal bests, 13 Canadian indoor records, 12 Canadian outdoor records, three Commonwealth records, and one world indoor record. We'd won three of the four short sprints against the powerful East Germans at the Eight Nations Meet, and more than 100 international medals in all.

For all of my athletes' achievements, I *knew* I had arrived when Chuck DeBus approached me in Cologne that season for advice about anabolic steroids.

DeBus had gotten his break in the business in the late 1970s at California State–Northridge, where he and another assistant coach, Bobby Kersee, helped develop a star-studded women's sprint group. (Among their top performers was Valerie Brisco-Hooks, who later won three gold medals at the 1984 Olympics.) DeBus told me that he had put members of his sprint group on six milligrams of stanozolol daily. The results were erratic, he complained. When his athletes had to lay off their steroids before the tested summer meets, they consistently crashed with sub-par performances.

When I asked DeBus about his cycling schedule, he replied that his athletes were on uninterrupted, steady-state doses throughout the season, except for required clearance periods. He said he had followed the steroid practices of the coach of a former world record-holder. According to DeBus, the coach gave the runner five milligrams of Dianabol every day throughout both training and competition, since steroids were not banned at the time.

Without referring specifically to my group, I advised DeBus how the East Germans cycled their Dianabol to avoid crashing. I thought little of the exchange at the time. It seemed no more than a professional courtesy, an analysis of the tools of our trade.

Pointing Toward Helsinki

As we entered the 1983 season, the International Olympic Committee finally addressed its second-biggest problem: the rules that governed amateurism. To that point, it had been technically prohibited for an athlete to accept any financial compensation beyond token expenses during a competition. The rules were absurd, hailing as they did from track and field's upper-class origins, when the sport was still a hobby for young white gentlemen. While meet promoters and the national and international federations reaped huge profits from ticket sales and television revenues, the stars of the show were expected to train full time for the pure love of competition. In practice, the amateur rules had been ignored since the 1920s. They accomplished two things: top athletes were forced to operate outside the rules, and meet directors—unbound by written contracts—found it easier to cheat the less established performers.

During my time at Stanford, assistant coach and former sportswriter Bud Spencer related a conversation he'd had with Charlie Paddock a half-century before. Paddock, the 1920 Olympic champion in the 100 metres, had told Bud he was clearing $500 a week at meets in Scandinavia, a princely sum in that era. Sonja Henie, the legendary Norwegian figure skater and three-time Olympic gold medallist, did even better. The night before each meet, her father invited the promoter to a poker game and told him how much he would lose. The father's luck never failed—and Sonja became one of the wealthiest amateurs of all time.

By the 1970s, it was commonplace to see athletes and agents lined up outside the door of an unmarked hotel room in a Grand Prix city, waiting to get paid by the meet promoter for their appearances. The ruling powers winked at this breach as long as the participants kept quiet about it. But in 1977, when Guy Drut, a French hurdler and defending Olympic champion, publicly admitted that he had accepted appearance fees, the IAAF banned him until 1981. For Drut's less candid associates, however, nothing changed.

Six years later, the bureaucrats gave in to reality. Athletes would now be allowed to establish trust funds where they could deposit endorsement earnings or appearance fees. While the funds were theoretically frozen until after the athletes retired, the new rules permitted periodic withdrawals for "living expenses"—and the loophole was liberal enough to put track's superstars behind the wheels of Porsches and Ferraris.

My sprinters weren't yet at that level, and their earning potential was limited by the small Canadian market. Nonetheless, I set about arranging endorsement contracts with Adidas. The amounts were quite low in 1983: about $500 a month for Angella, and $250 for Desai, Ben, Tony, and Mark. But they supplemented the athletes' meagre carding subsidies, kept food on their tables, and allowed them to train without the distraction of a part-time job. Over the next three years, I spent up to 30 hours a week seeking out financing for my runners. I accepted it as a necessary chore to keep my sprinters in the sport.

By the same token, I later refused to endorse a Canadian Track and Field Association drive to raise athletes' club membership fees to $1,000 and thereby pay the coaches, virtually all of whom were working as volunteers. The Optimist club had never collected more than $60 a year from its athletes, and Ross Earl and I agreed that we wouldn't start imposing high fees now. We weren't running a country club, after all. We maintained that the clubs should *generate* income for their athletes, not siphon money from them. If the coaches wanted to be paid, their clubs should seek out funds from other sources—from corporations, for example.

Our over-training caught up with Angella in 1983. Had she continued her rate of improvement that year, she might have become the world's top woman sprinter. But as she'd gotten faster, she'd also become more fragile—and I didn't yet know enough to cut her workload back. Her indoor season was ruined by thigh and groin injuries, which led to a chronic case of sciatica, a painful nerve condition. She received treatment that summer from an expert in Munich and improved temporarily, but was slow to regain top form, and capped her season by crushing her finger in a door hinge.

As Angella regressed, Desai advanced. He swept the nationals that summer, tied Harry Jerome's Canadian record for the 100 metres with a 10.17, and improved his 200 to 20.29.

Ben was making even more rapid progress. He won his first Grand Prix event in Munich, where he logged a new personal best of 10.19, the best time ever by a Canadian at sea level. Ben's starts, in particular, were the talk of the circuit; his eccentric form aside, no one could match him out of the blocks. Then, at the World Championships in Helsinki, his gift deserted him. He started poorly in his opening rounds and even worse in the semi-final, from which he failed to advance. He seemed to be panicking, which was out of character for Ben. After the semi, I sat him down for a long talk. We were joined by Don Quarrie, the veteran Jamaican star. Just as Hasely Crawford had tabbed Tony as the world's next great 100-metre man, and worked with him informally whenever he could, so Quarrie had taken Ben under his wing. (At 32, Quarrie was getting on in years, but he would still run well enough to win a silver on Jamaica's 4x100 relay team in the 1984 Olympics.) His mentor's relationship with Ben was genuinely selfless—a rare quality in the track world.

Ben told us he'd been concerned about his start for a number of reasons: his earlier problem in the preliminary heats; the headwind he'd be fighting; and—most of all—his perceived need to get out front because he knew the others would be outrunning him toward the end. *There* was the problem: The more you *try* to do something, the worse it will get. Quarrie sympathized with Ben's plight. In his own career, he said, he'd often found semi-finals more nerve-racking than finals, since you had to get past the semi to do anything at all in the big race. But Ben's anxiety was misplaced, he added: "You're already the best starter in the world—you *always* come out in front. The last thing you need to do is worry about how to get a better start." It was simple advice, but it helped. Ben would never have a starting slump again.

Ben was crazy about cars. Unfortunately, his limited and erratic income made it difficult for him to get financing to buy one. One day he asked me if I'd co-sign for an old Pontiac Trans Am he'd picked out. After I agreed, Tony began pestering me for the same favour. I asked Paul Poce, the Canadian distance coach, if I could co-sign for two different people at the same time. "Sure," Paul replied, "you can go to jail more than once." Despite this lack of reassurance, I helped Tony as well.

As Ben became more prosperous, his auto mania would wheel out of control. In the five years that followed the purchase of that first Pontiac, he would buy two Corvettes, a Toyota Supra, a Mazda 626 (for his mother), a Porsche 928, and, finally, a Ferrari Testarossa. I tried to discourage Ben from turning his cars over so quickly—his depreciation costs alone were huge—but he was stubborn, even compulsive on this score. He loved to go fast and in style, no matter the expense.

Carl Lewis had jolted the track world two months before Helsinki with his performance at the U.S. National Championships in Indianapolis. In his greatest feat ever, Carl ran the 200 metres in 19.75 seconds—just three hundredths off the world record, and *more than two tenths faster* than the previous best time at sea level. But what impressed observers most of all was the *way* he ran it. Lewis began waving his arms in celebration when he was 11 strides—a good 25 metres—from the finish line, which cost him at least two tenths and a certain record. Flying past the tape, he went on to complete the lap, with no visible fatigue, at a pace that might have won the 400 metres.

Fear and Testing in Caracas

Even as the IAAF adopted a more rational stance toward professionalism, it denied the reality of steroid use. The federation pronounced that drug testing would become mandatory at all major international meets, and that testosterone levels would be monitored in addition to steroids as of January 1, 1983. Injectable (either water-based or oil-based) testosterone had been popular since the steroid ban was instituted in 1975. For throwers and lifters, the hormone bridged any gap created by their steroid clearance times, enabling them to maintain their strength through their meets. For sprinters, testosterone was occasionally used as a supplement to synthetic steroids and growth hormone.

Since testosterone is found naturally in the body—in both men and women—a simple, qualitative test would not work. Instead, the testers set a maximum acceptable ratio of testosterone to epitestosterone of 6:1. (Epitestosterone is the epimer, or mirror image, of testosterone, and is generally found in the urine in equal measure to the male sex hormone. When testosterone is injected, it has a dual effect; it raises the body's testosterone level and lowers the epitestosterone level.) If an athlete's ratio exceeded the 6:1 maximum, it would be assumed that he or she had violated the ban.

The new era's acid test came at the inaugural World Championships in Helsinki in August 1983. (After two consecutive Olympic boycotts, it marked the first gathering of all the world's best track and field athletes since 1972.) But at the end of the meet, the IAAF's medical lab reported not a single positive finding, not even among the throwers.

Those who knew the performers at Helsinki could only become more cynical about the latest doping-control drive. One Eastern Bloc woman, an outstanding international runner, looked like a linebacker; even the East Germans made fun of her behind her back. A South Korean observer was particularly impressed by this leviathan among women.

"What that girl take?" the observer asked an official in the stands.

"I don't know, probably a lot of testosterone," the official replied.

"Oh, yeah?" said the Korean, cutting straight to the chase. "How much does it cost?"

Six years later, at the Dubin Inquiry, Manfred Donike, the IAAF lab director from West Germany, admitted that two athletes at Helsinki had tested above the accepted testosterone ratio, but claimed that no action was taken because the urine samples were too dilute. (When athletes drink large volumes of fluids before or after their events, their urine may become so diluted that lab tests cannot be reliably conducted; the proportion of chemical compounds—including banned substances—to water content is too low.) Richard Pound, vice-president of the International Olympic Committee, would testify at the Dubin Inquiry that he was "astounded" at the absence of positives at the meet.

How did the athletes survive the stepped-up battery of drug tests at Helsinki? In a jolting 1984 interview with *Runner's World*, Cliff Wiley, the American 400-metre man, claimed that there were "at least 38 people who were caught, who tested positive, and 17 or so were Americans. The problem was that their names were so big and there were so many of them that the organizers said, 'Hey, we're going to taint our Games. We're going to ruin the sport.'... So they didn't kick them out."

Wiley's charge—that the World Championships in Helsinki had been the scene of a "blanket type of amnesty"—seemed plausible in light of the debut made by the testosterone ratio test at that meet. According to research by Dr. Mauro DiPasquale, former chairman of the International Powerlifting Federation's medical committee, an associate professor of physical and health education at the University of Toronto, and an author who has compiled what is probably the world's largest data base on performance-enhancing drugs, it is especially tricky to gauge a safe clearance time for testosterone. When a male athlete injects the hormone, he depresses his body's own hormone production—to be precise, his hypothalamic-pituitary-testicular (HPT) axis. (Women react similarly via their hypothalamic-pituitary-ovarian axis.) The athlete's testosterone level may stay depressed for a time after the drugs are halted. But at some point—it could be days or even weeks later—his body will adjust to its withdrawal state. It will respond by manufacturing more endogenous (or natural) testosterone—often considerably more than it made before the injections began. This phenomenon, known as "rebound," can result in wildly fluctuating testosterone ratios long after any injections cease.

Consider these three actual cases, as cited by Dr. DiPasquale. In the first, an Italian stopped taking stanozolol injections 12 weeks before a tested meet; Dianabol tablets six weeks before; and testosterone propionate injections (which clear fastest) three weeks before. In each case, his clearance time would have been considered more than adequate. But to the thrower's dismay, his testosterone ratio was measured at 17:1—almost three times the permitted ceiling.

In the second case, a U.S. hammer thrower went off aqueous testosterone 10 days before a meet and Dianabol tablets three days before. The Dianabol was not detected, but he was tripped up by a testosterone level of 11:1.

In the third case, another American stopped taking aqueous testosterone only two days before the drug test and recorded a legal ratio of 2.5:1. Yet when the same athlete halted the same dose of testosterone a *week* before another test, his ratio was a positive 9:1.

In the period that preceded Helsinki in 1983, it stands to reason that athletes would be extra conservative in observing their clearance times, as they wouldn't know what to expect from the testosterone ratio test. I knew many athletes who used testosterone going into Helsinki, with clearance times ranging from 3 to 14 days. Given the rebound effect, the careful people may have been more vulnerable than the reckless ones—making it inconceivable that no one would test positive.

In late August, shortly after the World Championships, our team gathered by CTFA command for yet another major meet: the Pan Am Games in Venezuela. It was a mistake for us to go in the first place; most of our people had run too often that summer and were well past their peak. (We knew there was no use in objecting, however, since carded athletes are obligated by their contracts to compete in designated meets.) It became a worse mistake after our cut-rate plane fares entailed a 22-hour journey from Toronto to the meet site near Caracas, including a six-hour holdover in New York. Add in unsanitary dorms and execrable food, and it was no surprise when almost everyone came down with an intestinal bug. Molly Killingbeck lost 11 pounds in three days and had to be hospitalized. Infuriated, I moved the entire sprint team to the downtown Hilton (where the Canadian officials and swim team had been lodged in the first place), and paid the tab myself.

Paranoia was in the air. The hemisphere's athletes were terrified by reports that the Pan Ams would usher in a new era of sophisticated drug testing. American officials had touched off the panic by telling their people that the Pan Am lab equipment was unbelievably sensitive—that people could be caught up to three months after taking oral steroids, that the new machines could be calibrated to unheard-of sensitivities, and that the IAAF had flown in Manfred Donike, its resident anti-doping hard-liner. (West German performances fell off markedly after 1976 when Donike—dubbed by coaches as "the hunter"—initiated meet testing there.) According to Cliff Wiley, the 400-metre runner, "Our coaches warned everyone in Florida before we went down to Caracas, 'Don't go there unless you know you can pass this test.' And then they warned us again in Caracas, 'If you think you can't pass this test, tell us.' And then they helped them ship out."

Eleven U.S. athletes fled the Pan Ams, never to return. Nine other Americans stayed to play and were disqualified after positive tests, along with ten athletes from other countries.

Much of the panic came from misinformation. People were caught at the Pan Ams not by some revolutionary lab equipment, but because the old equipment was finally being used. (In a vain effort to quell the panic, Donike issued a public statement to that effect—that the testers had nothing new. It was a strange announcement from an official who should have been pleased to see drug users withdraw from the competition.) The snared athletes had simply come into the meet dirty—out of arrogance, out of past experience, out of the well-founded assumption that their opponents would be doing the same thing. I knew that a Canadian who tested positive, a weightlifter, had taken steroids up to two days before he competed. My own athletes, who had obeyed their standard clearance requirements, had no problems—although Desai was criticized in the American press after a quadriceps injury forced him to pull out of the 100-metre final, a ploy used by others to avoid a test.

The 1983 Pan Ams represented the largest drug scandal in track and field history—a time when the dope busters appeared to close ground on the dope takers. But the crackdown was limited and momentary. Even if the IAAF's technology had lived up to the rumours, even if the testers had been trying their hardest, the athletes would inevitably have regained their advantage. They could always find an untestable substance, some new variation on the testosterone molecule. There would always be a steroid gap.

The laissez-faire essence of international track and field was on display earlier that summer in Los Angeles, at a dual meet between the U.S. and G.D.R. national teams. (The Canadian team was in town for a separate competition, and we shared practice facilities with the G.D.R. at the University of Southern California.) The

East Germans won—a remarkable feat for a country of barely 16 million. They showcased a state-run system which left nothing to chance and which had vaulted their team to the very top. The G.D.R. sent 50 staff members to L.A. to accompany 80 athletes, including the personal coaches for each of their top competitors. Everyone was on time for every practice; the coaches weren't left standing around to wait for some prima donna.

But while I was impressed by the team's organization, I was thunderstruck by the size of its athletes. This was the first time I'd ever seen the East Germans at an untested venue—the national federations routinely notified one another in advance as to whether a meet would be tested—and the contrast was dramatic. (When going on or off Dianabol, an average sprinter's weight may fluctuate up to 10 to 12 pounds.) Marita Koch, their 100-metre star, was simply gigantic, with hamstrings that looked wider across than they were long, like those of a cat. Entry-mate Marlies Göhr, the world-record holder, was equally impressive. When Marlies tried on a pair of Angella's tights, presented as a gift, her thighs stretched the material to the limit—she was far larger than Angella, who was no pixie herself. (Marlies needed some cheering up. After she defeated Evelyn Ashford in the 100, Ashford stormed off and refused to come to the victory stand, and the medal presentation was cancelled.)

But the sprinters had nothing on the G.D.R.'s throwers, who were in their element at the USC weight room. With disconcerting nonchalance they hoisted everything they could lay their hands on, then dropped the iron plates to the floor until the concrete was cross-hatched with cracks. Even the svelte Petra Felke, a 130-pound javelin thrower, was booming up 205-pound snatch lifts—equal to my personal best as a 185-pound male in college. At the other extreme there was shot-putter Udo Beyer, the 1976 Olympic gold medallist, a cool six-foot-six and 330 pounds. He was doing effortless quarter squats with nine 45-pound plates on each end of a 45-pound bar—855 pounds in all—and the bar was bowing like the wings of a condor.

This was what we were up against, I thought. *This* was world-class track.

Udo's sister Gisela, a discus star, had come along as well, all six-foot-two and 250 pounds of her. Gisela was a friend of female shot-putter Ilona Slupianek, who was about five-eleven and 250, and had been suspended five years earlier for steroids—the only G.D.R. track and field athlete to be caught in 20 years of acknowledged, institutionalized doping there. (In 1980, Ilona staged a gold-medal comeback at the Moscow Olympics—a Games without a single positive drug test.) At one afternoon practice, a paunchy Canadian shot-putter named Marty Catalano padded out on the track, his training bag stuffed with roast beef sandwiches and a thermos of cappuccino. He unzipped his bag, set up his picnic, then took out his shot and began to warm up. Then Slupianek arrived. Without so much as a stretch she picked up a 16-pound men's shot (nearly twice the weight of the women's model), and threw it 17 metres—a distance Marty might reach on a good day. The Canadian watched silently for a moment, then picked up his sandwiches, zipped his bag, and left.

That evening I spied two of the G.D.R.'s female throwers on their way to the cafeteria for dinner. They were gotten up in frilly dresses with matching purses, and were perched on improbably flimsy high heels. In between the dresses and the shoes, one was reminded of why these women were here: their calves were like tree trunks, their Achilles tendons like bridge cables. A childhood memory flashed before me: the dancing hippos from *Fantasia*.

But the East Germans were no joke. In fact, they were a menace. They had gotten so strong that they'd outgrown the stadium. Three days before their meet, one of their javelin throwers let one fly and watched it in admiration—until he saw that it was heading straight for the high-jump pit, some 300 feet away on the far side of the in-field. "Look out!" he yelled, and the jumpers scattered to avert impalement. The javelin skipped off the pit—at a world-record distance or close to it—and sailed out beyond the high-jump apron. (Out of respect for the drug-linked progress in this event, and to protect athletes and spectators alike, the IAAF later modified the javelin so that it would nose-dive, shaving about 50 feet off the throwers' range.)

As the East German athletes practised, a troika of physiotherapists stood back to back to back in the middle of the in-field,
smoking cigarettes and gossiping, but always looking outward for
the slightest sign of injury: a triangle of vigilance. Two days before the dual meet, Udo Beyer twisted his ankle on the toe board at
the edge of the shot-put circle. The physios sprang into action like
a pit crew at the Indianapolis 500, kit bags in tow. Within seconds
they had numbed the ankle with an ethyl chloride spray and were
wrapping it to keep the swelling down.

The next day I ran into Udo and asked him how he was feeling.
"Oh yeah, we've got good doctors," he said. "I'll be ready, no
problem." He told me the physios had wrapped him so tight that
when they'd tried to drain the ankle that evening, the fluid from the
sprain had blown the aspiration needle right out of its plunger.

The day after that, Udo Beyer broke the world record.

Later that summer at Helsinki, where the East Germans performed
superbly once again, I renewed my acquaintance with Edwin
Tepper, the G.D.R.'s head sprint coach. I asked him if they planned
to prepare for the Olympics with any training camps in North
America. "No," he said, "we'll stay in the G.D.R. for all our
preparation, and then we'll come to L.A. and then—" He smashed
his fist into the other palm, loud enough to make me start.

From the people who brought you the blitzkrieg....

Toward the end of September, as it came time to regroup for the
new season, Desai had disappeared. He didn't show up for training,
and broke three appointments until I finally cornered him—to hear
him tell me that he'd lost faith in my training because he hadn't run
well at Helsinki. This made no sense to me. In 1983, after all, Desai
had set personal bests in the 100 (where he tied Harry Jerome's
Canadian record of 10.17) and in the 200, set a national record in the
indoor 300 metres, and made the final in the World Championships.
"But you panicked in Helsinki and tightened up—that's been your
weakness," I said, in an old refrain.

But Desai was adamant. He insisted that he wasn't strong enough, that he needed to train harder and lay a deeper base of endurance. My opinion was that people were leaving him behind at the end of the race not primarily because they were stronger (though they might have been), but because they were *faster* at their top velocity. It went back to my core tenet: It wouldn't do Desai any good to build stamina at 11 metres per second when he needed to go at least 11.5 metres per second to win the 100 against international competition—and about 12 metres per second to take aim at the world record. In the meantime, Desai needed above all to relax. If he ran his perfect race and Carl Lewis ran like Carl Lewis, Desai would still trail by two metres at the finish. There was nothing he could do about that—he had to let Lewis pull away, and tend to his own business. He needed enough confidence to *lose* and still run his best.

Desai had been my best male athlete almost from the start and now, just as the Olympic final lay within our sights, he was leaving. And so, predictably, was Mark McKoy, Desai's best friend on the team. Mark patterned his training after Desai, followed his pace in our special endurance runs, and now he would follow Desai out of our group as well.

I could claim but limited credit for Mark's progress as a hurdler; he was the most self-reliant athlete I'd ever met. I had no idea what he was doing about drugs, for example, although Angella had seen a bottle of testosterone in his bag at the 1981 World Cup trials. But while Mark's exit felt less like a desertion, it was a larger loss. He had placed fourth in the 110-metre hurdles in Helsinki, the best finish of any Canadian, and was a good bet to medal in Los Angeles. (As it turned out, Mark would run fourth there as well.)

Desai never found another coach. There was no place for him to go; he knew more about sprinting than anyone in Canada after Gerard and myself. The next several years would be hard for him. In 1983, he had won the nationals in the 100 and was the only Canadian to make the World Championship finals. In 1984, while training on his own, he would finish third in the nationals behind Ben and Tony, and would be the only one of the three *not* to make the Olympic final. We would eventually patch up our differences, but Desai's crisis of confidence would never be resolved.

New Protocols

My team's accomplishments brought me no special cachet among my peers in Canada. At a seminar I gave in the fall of 1983, one coach walked out in the middle. "Charlie's just got results because he has a bunch of niggers," he muttered. The sentiment was typical, if rarely expressed out loud.

On the matter of drugs there was little more enlightenment. Mike Mercer, now a shot and discus coach, forced the issue at the annual symposium of the Coaching Association of Canada. He stated that steroids were used extensively throughout the world and had inflated the Olympic qualifying standards that Canadian athletes were being pushed to meet. If Sport Canada didn't want people to use drugs, when would it adjust its standards to reflect reality? At that Richard Campion, director of the Canadian Weightlifting Federation, stood up and flatly declared that the Eastern Bloc athletes were "winning on the basis of superior training programs, not steroids." (This assertion would become all the more absurd in light of the 15 official positives that Canadian weightlifters would generate from 1983 to 1989.)

That ended the discussion. Mercer left the meeting shaking his head, and I saw no point in getting involved.

The psychology buffs were out in force at that conference. Everywhere I looked, a shrink was holding forth about "mental readiness" or some such blather. It occurred to me that Sport Canada knew that its athletes weren't prepared to win at that level and so it needed scapegoats—the athletes themselves. *It wasn't our fault*, the officials would say, after the fact. *God knows we did everything for them, but they just weren't psychologically tough enough.*

At the time, the Soviets and East Germans were mounting a no-holds-barred war in bobsledding technology. Both countries were spending up to a quarter-million dollars apiece for their sleds, while the Canadians were bumbling along in $12,000 used models that the Swiss team had discarded. The toughest minds in the world would be hopelessly outclassed in those junkers. "Look, this is ridiculous," I finally told the symposium. "If you want to win Le Mans, you go out and buy a Porsche 956. You don't get a soapbox derby car with rope steering and put a psychologist in the back to tell you how to drive the damn thing."

I wasn't always at odds with officialdom. One afternoon in 1983, Senator Ray Perrault of Vancouver, Canada's newly designated minister for fitness and amateur sport, showed up at our track unannounced. "They said you're the guy producing the results in amateur sport," he told me, "so I thought I should talk to you." We spent the rest of the day together before he asked me for a ride—to catch a subway. Perrault was my kind of minister—no-nonsense, unpretentious, eager to learn. Unfortunately, he was shuffled out of office a few months later and lost his chance to make an impact.

I also liked the hard-working Otto Jelinek, one of Perrault's successors. But I found that even the best politicians couldn't get past the permanent government—the technocrat advisers with a vested interest in the status quo.

As we pointed toward the 1984 season, we needed a doctor— someone who could treat problems like Angella's sciatica and also oversee the drug protocols. As it stood, the athletes were visiting various physicians for blood tests, a scattershot system at best. I wanted more control and more reliable feedback; any mistake could be terribly costly, even irrevocable. I didn't want to repeat the lesson of Alexis Paul-MacDonald, an Optimist sprinter (though not in my group) who had been suspended in 1981 after testing positive for anabolics. To the end, Alexis insisted that she had never touched steroids, and that the positive had been triggered by her use of the Pill, which had a similar molecular structure. (Although the IAAF denied her appeal, it took the problem seriously enough to attempt to ban certain birth control pills.)

In October 1983, on a referral from a chiropractor we used, I accompanied Angella to see Dr. Jamie Astaphan, a St. Kitts native who'd received his medical degree from the University of Toronto and was known for his skillful treatment of sports injuries. Astaphan was refreshingly jovial and easy-going, and he impressed me by spending 90 minutes on Angella's medical history and current difficulties. While he knew little about track per se, his diagnostic skills were immediately apparent. He examined Angella before being told anything about her sciatica—and quickly confirmed the conclusions of two prominent doctors she'd seen previously that summer.

While Astaphan acknowledged his inexperience with performance-enhancing drugs, he was willing to learn more and to steer us through the pharmaceutical shoals. The state of steroid use had grown far more complex than it had been even five years before, when Dianabol was still predominant. Athletes were now trying a wide range of steroids and other performance-enhancing substances. By using frontier drugs, they were able to stay ahead of the tests; the IAAF's computerized equipment could flag a suspect metabolite only if specifically programmed to do so. With this new generation of pharmaceuticals, it was no longer possible to tell who was "on" by simply gauging their muscularity; a user could as easily be lean as bulging. We had entered a brave new world of designer drugs, and there was no turning back.

Shortly after seeing Astaphan, Angella visited Dr. Robert Kerr, a Los Angeles sports physician who was famous for his ministrations to a sizeable portion of the U.S. Olympic team. Kerr believed that Anavar worked more effectively for women than Dianabol, and directed Angella to take five milligrams per day. He also prescribed an injectable drug that had become the rage in elite track circles: human growth hormone, a pituitary extract which was used therapeutically in cases of dwarfism. Where steroids acted primarily on muscles, growth hormone strengthened bones and tendons as well.

When I first read the monograph insert, I got excited: Growth hormone would begin to break down fat in the body *within 20 minutes* of administration; it would enhance protein synthesis and increase the proportion of lean body mass; it had no known side effects. Best of all, the drug was not on the banned list. (Though banned today, it still cannot be detected, since no test can distinguish between the hormone made by the athlete's body and that introduced by syringe.) Despite the hormone's high price—$150 for a one-week's supply—it seemed to hold spectacular promise.

As a further supplement, Kerr also recommended two amino acids, arginine and ornithine, and a synthetic amino acid called L-dopa, which is used to treat Parkinson's disease. All three substances increased the body's secretion of growth hormone, and none was banned.

When this protocol was laid before Astaphan in Toronto, he deferred to Kerr's expertise while pledging to continue his own research. He later advised that we delete L-dopa (which caused stiffness) and substitute Dixarit, a drug used therapeutically to treat high blood pressure. In the spring of 1984, Astaphan advised us to include an injectable mix of vitamin B12 and inosine (a non-steroidal anabolic), neither of them banned, and occasional small doses of aqueous testosterone. He obtained all of these for us and never billed us in full, as he knew that our means were limited.

After detailed consultations with Astaphan, Angella, Ben, and Tony employed this expanded protocol (with the two men staying on Dianabol rather than Anavar) at their training camp that March in Guadeloupe. The athletes injected one another, as I was squeamish about needles and hoped to avoid them if I could.

Despite the complexity of our new drug program, it remained conservative by U.S. standards. I would later learn that one group of American women was using three times as much growth hormone as Kerr had suggested, in addition to 15 milligrams per day of Dianabol, another 15 milligrams of Anavar, large amounts of testosterone, and thyroxine, the synthetic thyroid hormone used by athletes to speed the metabolism and keep people lean. (While research has yet to prove that "stacking" several steroids provides any greater anabolic effect than using a single drug, anecdotal evidence suggests that it may.) The group was additionally taking a variety of stimulants, including amphetamines and strychnine.

The Americans also surpassed us at the federation level. Sport Canada and the Canadian Olympic Association issued stern anti-drug admonitions on the one hand, then set forbidding Olympic qualifying standards on the other—standards that were impossible to reach without drugs. (Heading into the 1980 Olympics, the initially proposed COA standard for the women's 1,500 metres was *faster* than the world record at the time—a wildly optimistic projection.) The U.S. Olympic Committee was considerably more helpful to its athletes. Beginning early in 1984, the USOC sponsored an "educational," non-punitive testing program at the IOC-accredited lab at UCLA. Officially, the program was designed to familiarize Americans with dope-testing procedures. In effect, it allowed U.S. athletes to cut their clearance times to the bone—a huge home-court advantage. (As might be expected from such trial-and-error experimentation, up to 50 percent of these tests reportedly came up positive.)

The accepted clearance time for oral steroids, for example, was 21 days. But one male thrower found he could pass a test seven days after his last daily dose of 85 milligrams of oral Dianabol. And American women discovered they could pass only *three* days after their last dose of Anavar (an elusive steroid to test for) or Winstrol. In Los Angeles, American athletes would come into the Olympic Games at their drug-supported best.

The Bronze

As we approached the 1984 Olympics, I was pleased with our prospects. Our relay teams were definite medal contenders. Carl Lewis was in a league by himself in the men's sprints; he'd been ranked first in the 100 metres, without serious challenge, since 1981. But no one else was demonstrably better than Ben, who had opened the season with an impressive 10.21 and seemed to be gaining by the day. Angella was training better than ever, to the point where I thought she might run in the 10.90s and possibly win. Evelyn Ashford, the U.S. champion who'd run a world record 10.79 at altitude in 1983, had hurt her hamstring twice already that season and might be coming in at less than her best. In addition, the Communist boycott had removed perennial adversary Marlies Göhr. It looked as if the gold medal was up for grabs.

(Göhr was no happier about the 1984 boycott than Angella had been in 1980; just as the U.S. had arm-twisted Canada out of the Moscow Olympics, so had the Soviet Union pressured a reluctant East Germany to pass up Los Angeles. Göhr evinced her displeasure during the 4x100-metre relay at the "Friendship Games" in Moscow that summer, the Eastern equivalent of the 1980 "Freedom Games." As the G.D.R. anchor, Göhr was leading the

142

race when she stopped 50 yards short of the tape, hurled her baton into the stands, and stomped off the track.)

But the CTFA seemed determined to kill our chances. The murder weapon was the Canadian National Championships that June, which would double as our Olympic trials. The meet had been committed to Winnipeg years before, but preparations for a new track surface there had fallen behind schedule. When the surface wasn't laid in 1983, I knew we were in deep trouble; given Winnipeg's late spring, there was no way the track would be cured and ready by June. I voiced my concern to the CTFA: that an uncured track would provoke a rash of injuries as the athletes struggled over the spongy surface. The only sensible measure, I said, was to move the nationals elsewhere. It became clear, however, that political and financial considerations outweighed our athletes' welfare. "I don't care if they run on *dirt*," blustered Tom MacWilliam, the CTFA's technical director. "They're going to run in Winnipeg."

In the end, the athletes ran in Winnipeg, and many of them—both mine and other coaches'—got hurt. Ben logged a wind-aided 10.01 to win the 100, but strained his hamstring in the process. Angella injured her quadriceps in the 200, and Molly Killingbeck, our 400-metre national champion, suffered a quad pull which appeared to have ruined her chance to run in the Olympics, now just four weeks away.

We returned to Toronto, where Dr. Astaphan worked a minor miracle. Upon examination of Molly's leg, Astaphan found a hole where the muscle had been partially torn from the tendon— a severe injury which normally required at least two months to heal. Astaphan prescribed complete rest for five days, along with electronic muscle stimulation and a medication called Varidase. He also recommended that Molly return to train at short distances before building up to the 400 metres that she would run with our relay team in Los Angeles, as opposed to the conventional tack of starting long and then building speed. Four weeks later, Molly ran her relay leg in a personal best.

I had mixed feelings about the 1984 Olympics. The Americans' hyper-nationalism was certainly obnoxious, and the warm-up area at the Olympic stadium was grossly inadequate. A few strips of fenced-in lawn gave the scores of sprinters barely enough room to stretch, and practice starts were out of the question. At the same time, I had to admire the efficiency and splendour of the show in Los Angeles. In contrast to the government incompetence that stained the 1976 Olympics in Montreal (and cost Canadian taxpayers more than a billion dollars), the 1984 Games were underwritten by private sponsors and actually turned a profit.

The Optimists' performances were mixed as well. Angella ran her first heat in a smooth 11.23 and appeared headed toward a competitive 11-flat. But she strained her hamstring in the quarter-final, and even Super Mike couldn't put her back together again within 24 hours. Her semi-final the next day was stacked with five good runners, which meant that she couldn't jog her way through to the final, since only four would qualify. Angella survived that test, but her muscle let go toward the finish. Heavily taped and limping, she finished last in the final in 11.62. Just as in Helsinki, her body had betrayed her when it counted most. But this failure hit even harder; it summoned up the ghost of Moscow and all that might have been four years before. Evelyn Ashford had recovered enough to win the final in an Olympic record 10.97—a time within Angella's potential had she been sound.

Ben and Tony both made it to the men's 100-metre final, the first time two Canadians had gone that far. But Ben cramped his hamstring—at the site of his Winnipeg injury—in the semi. There was no new injury, but the muscle was very tight. Super Mike worked on him feverishly during the 90-minute intermission before the final, and Ben seemed to be all right. Then he false-started, a particular disadvantage for a top starter like Ben. Since a second false start would disqualify him, he would have to hold back, and he reacted poorly to the next gun. Normally ahead of the field after 10 metres, Ben was running fifth and well behind the pace-setter, the American Sam Graddy. At 50 metres, however, Ben surged. He took the lead at 80 metres, inches ahead of the fast-closing Lewis—the farthest Ben had ever led Carl to that point. It was then that Winnipeg came back to haunt us. Ben's leg cramped again. Lewis blew by him, as we'd expected, on his way to a fine time of 9.99 and a winning margin of 10 feet. (Films of the race show that the entire field was struggling over those last 20 metres—except for Carl, who maintained perfect form to the final stride.)

Over the last few metres, Graddy came on to finish second in 10.19, while Ben held on for third in 10.22. It was a mild disappointment, since Ben had been headed for the silver. On the other hand, an Olympic bronze was a giant step for a runner who'd finished in the top three in a Grand Prix event only once in his life, when he'd won Munich the year before.

My runners came through in the relays. Our men's 4x100-metre team, composed of Ben, Tony (who'd finished eighth in the 100-metre final), Desai, and Sterling Hinds, won the bronze. The Canadian women did even better, with both the 4x100 team (including the injured Angella) and the 4x400 squad taking silver medals. The latter team included three of my athletes: Charmaine Crooks, Jillian Richardson, and the recovered Molly Killingbeck. But our people were no match for the Americans, who swept the ten sprint events at these Olympics. The U.S. men set two Olympic records and one world mark. The U.S. women surprised everyone by breaking Olympic records in four of their five sprint events, and narrowly missing the fifth. Their improvement was most conspicuous in the 4x400 women's relay. In Helsinki, we had beaten the American women in this event. In Los Angeles, the Canadian women dramatically improved their Helsinki time and set a new Commonwealth record—yet the U.S. beat us by nearly three seconds.

In the wake of the U.S. Olympic Committee's non-punitive testing program, no Americans were exposed by drug tests at the Games. Of 14 foreign Olympic athletes who officially tested positive at Los Angeles, the most prominent victim in track and field was Martti Vainio, who lost his silver medal in the 10,000 metres and added to the doping legends among Finnish distance runners. Vainio's Olympic predecessor from Finland, a virtual unknown named Kaarlo Maaninka, had won the silver in the same event in 1980. Maaninka later admitted to blood doping—an untestable practice in which blood is withdrawn from the body and banked for later use. In the interim, the sample is centrifuged, a process which removes any steroid metabolites along with the blood plasma, leaving "clean" red cells to be reinjected shortly before the athlete's event. The benefit of blood-doping is substantial; an athlete's oxygen-carrying capacity may be expanded by as much as 10 to 15 per cent. (This practice was not banned by the IOC until after the 1984 Olympics—and after several members of the U.S. cycling team, including a number of Olympic medallists, admitted to doping with blood from outside donors.)

According to one theory, Vainio had been mistakenly doped with red cells still tainted by some metabolites of the steroid Primobolan—he'd been done in by his own blood. It seemed less likely that he might simply have erred in his protocol, given the Finnish Olympic Committee's documented history of doping education. In a letter dated June 18, 1976, the committee stated that it had no time to deal with "the moral side of the issue," but advised its athletes to consider the "practical advice" that committee doctors had obtained from "experts in the field." A brief treatise followed with details on clearance times.

The Los Angeles Olympics marked Ben's arrival on the international scene, as *Track & Field News* would acknowledge when it ranked him fourth in the 100 metres at the end of 1984. It would be some time, however, before Ben's reputation (and marketability) caught up with his performance. For one thing, there was widespread confusion over the meaning of a medal in the 1984 Olympics, given the Soviet Bloc's boycott. In women's swimming, for example, a bronze medal might be meaningless, as all the top competitors had sat out the Games. But in the men's 100 metres, the medals could not be devalued, since none of the missing Eastern Europeans had made the finals in Helsinki in 1983. Ben had faced the best sprinters in the world—period.

Nonetheless, Ben remained less than a hot item on the Grand Prix circuit immediately after the Olympics. In places like Brussels, which put on a "high-end" show with a handful of celebrity athletes, the meet directors were happier without him. They'd pay well into five figures for a marquee name like Carl Lewis, and somewhat less for a well-known, second-magnitude star—Calvin Smith, perhaps—who could go fast enough to keep the pace honest. The rest of the lanes would be filled by local heroes and nonentities, people who would be happy to run for free. A young comer like Ben didn't fit into this equation; his presence wouldn't sell any tickets that Lewis hadn't sold already, but his appearance fee would cut into the director's profit margin.

The sole exception was Zurich, where an insurance executive named Andreas Brügger strove to put on the most spectacular show in the world, and the balance sheet be damned. Brügger's meet was the best because he invited *every* star. World-class results were guaranteed. No matter who faltered, someone else was bound to come through. The Zurich *Weltklasse* might net less money than other meets, but it went unchallenged for prestige value; a win there meant more than at any other meet outside the Olympics or World Championships.

While Brügger was happy to give Ben a chance in August of 1984, he wasn't about to treat the young Canadian as one of the established royalty of the sport. While Lewis, Calvin Smith, and European record holder Marian Woronin were advanced straight to the final, Ben had to run in a preliminary heat to earn one of the five remaining lanes. Given the high level of competition, Ben had to go all out in his heat, and his muscles were tighter than we would have liked. For all that, he had a good start and a great middle surge in the final; Lewis could not begin to match his speed until 60 metres into the race, by which point Ben led the American by four feet. Ben held his lead through 94 metres—and then he broke a sacred rule. He looked back in wonder: *Where was Lewis?* The answer was just off his left hip, and then, in a blink, more than a metre ahead of him at the finish. Lewis ran 9.99 again, trailed by Harvey Glance in 10.09. Ben finished third in 10.12—a new Canadian record, even though he'd fallen apart at the end.

Although Zurich represented Lewis's sixth straight victory over Ben, dating back to 1980, there were signs that the streak might not last forever. Ben had shown he was capable of a 10.06 if he maintained his equilibrium. He had halved the gap between himself and Lewis from eight feet to four feet in one year. And if past progress was any guide, we could expect Ben to improve by another six hundredths in the coming season, whereas Lewis appeared to be levelling off.

During the three-week break I allowed my sprinters before we resumed training in September, Ben volunteered for some homework with his VCR. He studied several tapes of Lewis's best races, including Los Angeles, to see where the American was beating him. Ben concluded that Lewis had one critical advantage: The American was able to stay relaxed throughout the race and thus to hold form to the end. As he watched those races over and over, Ben realized just how close he was to reaching the top. A bit more confidence and a touch more strength, and he might be there.

Few were yet aware of it, but the greatest rivalry in the history of track's primal event was about to begin.

Conquering Heroes

Canada's track team won 14 medals—including eight by my runners, not including Desai—in Los Angeles in 1984, our best Olympic showing in more than 50 years. In a new spirit of optimism, CTFA executives concocted a document they called *Project 2000*, a journey into science fiction which envisioned Canada as the world's premier track and field power by the end of the millennium.

But a plan like that would take money, and lots of it. In 1984, we had succeeded *despite* the low level of government support. The CTFA's budget for competitions and related expenses, as set by Sport Canada, was a paltry $860,000—about 4 percent of Italy's. It was with great anticipation, then, that we awaited Sport Canada's response to the 1985 budget request made by Gerard Mach, now the CTFA's high-performance program director.

Gerard didn't receive his answer until April 1985. To reward our achievements of the year before, Sport Canada was *cutting* the CTFA's competitive budget by more than half, to $380,000. As Gerard gave me the bad news, he was sputtering with indignation. "Sport Canada says, 'Give us a plan,'" he said, "so I spend two months preparing my report. I ask for the *minimum* that any country needs to run a proper program—with an A-team, a B-team, and a junior team—and it's four million dollars. And they say, 'Ah, Gerard, we're very impressed, it's an excellent plan. Here's $380,000.' *Thank* you! I take my plan and I throw it in the trash!

"How am I supposed to work with a budget like that? *Project 2000*—they must be talking about $2,000, because that's what they'll be giving us by then!"

Sport Canada's budget cut would have serious and lasting repercussions. It made long-term goals meaningless, since the new generation of junior athletes—people who might have had just as much talent as Ben or Angella—would never get the same chance to succeed. There would be fewer warm-weather training camps to save runners' legs after long winters on hard indoor tracks; fewer competitions for the experience that every young athlete needs; less money for the European tours where my top people had come of age. The last would be especially crippling for our non-carded athletes, who needed overseas meets to spur them to better performances. Their only other avenue was to enter early-season meets in the United States. But these competitions were less beneficial, since American athletes held a formidable advantage in spring training because of their warmer climate—especially in the Sun Belt states, where most of the university track powers were located.

As a result, our younger athletes would have to compete almost exclusively at home, in cold weather, and on second-rate surfaces. They were further hindered by how our local meets were administered. In the United States and Europe, the national federations helped their own athletes perform at their best levels. They arranged for sprints to be run with tailwinds and for events to go off on time, to allow for orderly warm-ups. When athletes aimed for a big performance, whether to break a national record or to reach an Olympic standard, they usually encountered the best possible conditions. (There was less flexibility at major international or invitational meets. Since the most expensive seats were sold in advance near the sprints' finish line, meet officials couldn't shift the line at the last minute for the sake of a tailwind.)

In Canada few such efforts were made. At one open competition in Etobicoke, the athletes were forced to run into an *11-metre-per-second* gale—a wind so strong that hurdlers couldn't even reach the next hurdle in the normal three steps. At another Ontario competition, the events lagged five hours behind schedule. Under such conditions it was impossible for people to meet Sport Canada's ever more stringent carding requirements.

Five or ten years earlier, Optimist founder Ross Earl might have picked up the slack and helped to subsidize some of these younger athletes. But because of Sport Canada's reduced support, Ross still had to contribute toward travel and training camp expenses for our high-level performers. The Scarborough bingo revenues were stretched thin, and there was little left over for promising newcomers. And my services were stretched as well. With more than 20 senior athletes, all of whom required individual attention, I was unable to take on new people after the fall of 1984. To keep the sprint centre flourishing, I needed at least two full-time paid assistant coaches; I had but a single volunteer who showed up after his regular job. It did little good for my developing and junior athletes to travel with me and my top A-card runners. To find the right level of competition, these less advanced athletes needed a separate circuit. But I had no money for their tours (the meet promoters would pay expenses only for our best people) and no full-time coaches to travel with them.

As a result, many developing sprinters were driven from the sport by neglect. It became clear that there would be no new crop to replace my stars after they retired. Like any pyramidal structure, our nation's high-performance program would either grow or die—and Sport Canada had decreed that it would not grow.

My sprinters were slightly better off than most, since they'd been able to supplement their carding money (now a maximum of $650 a month) with small sponsorship stipends from Adidas and minor appearance fees from the Grand Prix circuit. But we were plunged into financial crisis in the fall of 1984 when our Adidas contracts were cancelled, with no prior notice from either the company or the CTFA. (We learned of the cancellation in the newspapers.) I later discovered that Don Fletcher and Glen Bogue, the CTFA's athlete services manager, had negotiated a modified arrangement with the company at a secret meeting to which Gerard Mach was not invited. The new deal preserved funding to the association (which would order the athletes to wear Adidas-supplied uniforms at the televised national championships), at the expense of monthly payments to my athletes—the ones who had generated the top performances that Adidas cared about. (Our athletes were vulnerable because they'd been the first to register their trust funds above board with the CTFA, as called for by international rules. Many of Canada's distance runners, by contrast, continued to conceal their financial arrangements and to receive their money under the table, and so were untouched by the association's coup.)

Instead of searching out new revenues for its bureaucratic needs, the CTFA had taken what little private funding my athletes had been able to garner. It was the worst time for my sprinters to be cut off, since sponsors are scarce during post-Olympic years. As a result, I spent an increasing amount of time—about half my work week in 1985—rustling up small endorsement contracts. Ben managed to recoup with a $450 monthly deal with Timex and later re-signed with Adidas, while Angella received a smaller amount from a manufacturer of protective rubber heel supports. She was running poorly that winter and more than once became dizzy in the starting blocks at practice. In January of 1985 she told me that she and Tony Issajenko were going to have a baby. After her series of disappointments on the track, she seemed happy to be taking a year off.

While I still had a dozen world-class runners in training, the old gang wasn't what it used to be. Desai and Mark were gone; Tony was increasingly hampered by his Achilles and other injuries; Angella was pregnant. I had only one international star remaining—but Ben Johnson would soon be providing all the excitement I needed.

With a year of observation and research under his belt, Dr. Astaphan was ready to take charge of our drug program for the 1985 season.

He took Ben and Tony off growth hormone, which he thought was overrated except as a means of speeding recovery from injuries. He also substituted a water-based, injectable version of Dianabol, which he deemed more effective than the Dianabol tablets we'd used previously. Since the doctor would administer the steroid injections himself in his Toronto office, along with shots of vitamin B12 and inosine, he retained more control than if he'd handed each sprinter a bottle of pills.

Astaphan's most important innovation was to alter the timing of our drug cycles. In previous seasons, my sprinters would train for up to eight weeks in the fall before beginning their drug regimen; the steroids were designed to boost the athletes' training capacity only *after* they'd fallen into a deep fatigue state. This made no sense to Astaphan. "Why dig yourself into a hole before you start the steroids?" he said. "Why not go with the steroids first, and start training from a position of strength?"

We adopted the new schedule and found that it helped our people peak earlier in the season—a definite plus, assuming that we could maintain that peak into the biggest meets. (This approach was antithetical to that of other Canadian coaches, whose athletes would not be trained to peak before mid-summer, but was clearly in line with the programs and performances of many of the world's leading sprinters.) Since my athletes avoided those early training overloads, they needed less of the steroids—and for shorter durations—than their competitors. And since our runners would be completing their steroid cycles earlier as well, they'd be less likely to run afoul of a drug test.

To head off any injuries, I closely monitored my sprinters throughout their speed work. If I spotted the slightest deterioration in form—if, for example, I heard Ben's feet strike a bit heavier on the track—I stopped him immediately and either moved him to a different training component or called it a day. To support my visual observations, I peppered my people with questions: How were they feeling? Was that last repetition more difficult than the one before? I would avoid, however, that old coach's favourite: *Can you do another one?* There is only one answer to a question like that: *Yes, I can.* Athletes will ignore their own instincts to please their coach. But I didn't want them to train harder; I wanted them to train smarter. I re-examined every drill. If I couldn't find a good reason for keeping it, it disappeared.

I made two other major changes in my coaching for 1985. (They were my last systematic revisions; day-to-day adjustments aside, the training program that would carry us to Seoul was now complete.) After toying with the idea for several years, I now had my runners develop their maximum velocity over *short* distances when speed training commenced in the fall, and then gradually stretch out at that top speed. I believed that stamina was important, *but only at a given velocity.* It is easier for sprinters to add distance at a set speed than to step up their speed at a set distance of 200 or 300 metres. With younger sprinters, the wrong kind of endurance work can cramp their potential. Since the body adapts to the work demanded of it, too many long runs at an intermediate velocity may convert undifferentiated (or "transitional") muscle fibres to red (slow-twitch) rather than white (fast-twitch), the raw material that sprinters need.

Like all modern sprint coaches, I restricted endurance work at the outset of a season, and began assigning speed work no later than four weeks into their training. I never wanted my runners to get too far away from our primary pursuit: more speed. After Ben had run a 10.12 in August of 1984, it made no sense for him to lose that speed through cross-country work. Instead, I sought to consolidate his gains and build on his performances from one year to the next. But most Canadian coaches continued to push numbing amounts of endurance work to build "a great base." And so they did—*but there was nothing on top of the base.* If these people had designed the Great Pyramid, it would have covered 700 acres and topped off at 30 feet. Their athletes were champions of the sand hills and the forest paths, but not of the sprints.

My second major modification involved our weight training, which we'd begun in 1980. Throughout 1984 I'd followed the lifting theories of Tudor Bompa, a former Romanian coach who now taught at York University. In the fall of 1985, however, I decided to adapt our strength work to my general training philosophy—that less was more. In my experience, larger muscles were more vulnerable to pulls and tears; my sprinters had become so strong that overload and injury were constant dangers. Just as I'd tailored our speed drills for high intensity but low volume, I now did the same for our lifting. Since we weren't aiming to bulk up (too much body mass might get in a sprinter's way), I pared our weight program to a few basic exercises which could challenge a high percentage of muscle groups with relatively few lifts. Total repetitions were cut by about 40 percent. In particular, I did away with the calf exercises favoured by Bompa. In my view, the Eastern Europeans overrated the importance of calf and ankle strength. Biomechanical analysis had shown that a sprinter generated seven times as much power at the hip as at the ankle. And if the calves became too large relative to the thighs, they would retard the runner's stride frequency, just as a metronome slows as its weight slides further from its fulcrum.

I also eliminated the traditional "conversion phase" which sprint coaches had adopted to bring velocities in weight-lifting closer to sprint speeds. I concluded that a sprinter's extremities moved so much faster in running than in lifting that any increase in lifting speed was irrelevant.

As my top sprinters progressed and became stronger, I sought guidance from Bishop Dolegiewicz, Canada's national shot-put record holder. More than anyone else around, Bishop knew the demands and dangers of high-intensity lifting. In contrast to Bompa, Bishop would never test himself for a new maximum with a single repetition; at the loads he was lifting (a 600-pound bench press, for example), he'd be inviting injury. Instead, he recommended that athletes escalate their work as they felt they were able, but not to risk a heavier load unless they could do at least two repetitions.

Bishop's long recovery periods—he rested up to 14 days between full-scale, maximum-intensity sessions—were especially controversial. But I was immediately receptive to his approach, since it dove-tailed with Horst Hille's 10-day tapers and Gerard's 10-day recovery periods after central nervous system overload. My runners became visibly fresher once I started following Bishop's advice. Everything was beginning to fit together.

My final revision was to have my athletes maintain their weight training throughout the entire season. Most sprint coaches would administer weight work in the fall and spring but cut it off during the summer competition period, for fear that they'd be sapping their athletes' strength. Their concern was legitimate, but it backfired. Since pure power is both the easiest component to gain *and* to lose, their runners would grow weaker soon after they stopped lifting. To avoid this deterioration, my athletes maintained low-volume lifting to within a few days of the biggest meets. At the same time, I understood that weight training was only a means to an end. If I saw that someone was drained from speed work, I would defer the sprinter's weight work to another day.

Of all my athletes, Ben was now the most powerful. In five years he had increased his bench press from 180 to 365 pounds—more than double his body weight of 160—with no end in sight. (Tony Sharpe, who was significantly larger than Ben, bench-pressed 320 pounds.) I'd known for years that Ben was immensely strong. His grip could be painfully firm (a good clue to an athlete's general strength, since few people train their grip), and he could pin anyone he rough-housed or wrestled with.

In Los Angeles in 1984, Ben was playing pool at the Olympic Village when he realized that his identity card—the required pass to all facilities—was missing. He searched the room, increasingly upset, then spotted a corner of the card protruding from the pants pocket of Lennox Lewis, the Canadian super-heavyweight boxer who would go on to win the gold medal at Seoul. After Ben made it aggressively plain that he wasn't pleased about the practical joke, Lewis responded by clamping him in a headlock. Ben proceeded to flip the 225-pound boxer over his shoulder and onto the pool table, ripping the joker's shirt in the process. Lewis backed off. "The guy is *crazy*," he muttered.

At the warm-up track later that day, I found Ben with an ice pack on his neck, which he'd strained in the ruckus. I suggested that if he wanted to embark on a boxing career, he might do better to start with the middleweights and work his way up.

Ben served notice of good things to come during the 1985 indoor season. At an invitational meet in Osaka, Japan, he set a new Canadian record of 6.56 in the 60 metres, just two hundredths off Houston McTear's world record. After a 20-hour plane trip to Paris, he came back two nights later to beat Sam Graddy in the World Indoor Championships. (Ben was so tired that he was sitting on the warm-up track 40 minutes before the 60-metre final. I came over and said, "Ben, it's time to warm up." "Warm up?" he replied. "I can't even *stand* up.")

We launched Ben's outdoor season at a May 11th meet in Modesto, California, against Carl Lewis, who had already been racing outdoors for weeks. (We didn't mind conceding the advantage, since we had no inkling that Ben might have a shot at the number-one ranking that year.) Carl won the race in the year's world-best time of 9.98, while Ben finished third in 10.16, a strong showing for a season's debut.

Once again we'd underestimated Ben's rate of improvement. In July, at a high-altitude meet, Ben ran a personal-best 10-flat. But Cecil Smith, the CTFA's records chairman, refused to recognize the performance as a Commonwealth and Canadian record because the meet was not sanctioned by TAC. Smith had complained for years about altitude-assisted performances, but when Ben ran a 10.04 after a poor start at the World Cup trials in Puerto Rico two months later, there could be no argument: Both records were his. ("Is this low enough for you?" Gerard taunted Smith after the race. "The ocean's right over there.")

And then, at the World Cup in Canberra, Australia, a meet where Carl Lewis was absent, Ben broke through once more, with a gold medal and a time of 10-flat into an 0.4-metre wind—the fastest time ever run into a headwind, and another Canadian and Commonwealth record. Best of all, the race demonstrated that Ben was capable of running a 9.95 under neutral conditions.

Lewis had met Ben earlier that year for a showdown at the Zurich *Weltklasse* in August. Carl had beaten Ben in seven straight matches, but the quadruple gold medallist suddenly appeared vulnerable. Lewis had been fighting a hamstring injury since May. He'd also been distracted by his business interests, from a Grammy Awards appearance to a record album he'd cut in Japan. He had to be anxious after Ben ran a 10.11 heat into another headwind. In the final, Ben's start was mediocre, but he came on quickly to go neck-and-neck with Calvin Smith for the lead. There would be no panicking this time; a year had made all the difference. Ben now had the strength to hold his form to the finish. He won the race in 10.18—a more than respectable time, considering that the wind had stiffened since his heat. Smith finished second in 10.19, Desai third in 10.26, and Carl well back in fourth at 10.31.

The king wasn't dead, but his throne had begun to teeter.

The final contest between Ben and Carl that year would be off the track, within the offices of *Track & Field News*, where the editors determined the sport's annual world rankings, including the paper coronation of the world's fastest human in the 100 metres. In retrospect, entering Ben at Modesto had been a strategic error. Along with a meaningless race in Cologne (both rivals were off form and lost to Woronin, but Carl had edged Ben, 10.27 to 10.29), Modesto gave Lewis a two-to-one edge for the year, as well as the season's best time of 9.98. On the other side, Ben had won the year's two most important races, in Canberra and Zurich, and his 10-flat in the World Cup was unquestionably the best 100-metre *performance* in 1985, given the conditions. There was also the question of Lewis's failure to run in Australia: Had he ducked the race to avoid another loss to Ben (as the American coach Russ Rogers had suggested to me), or had he been squeezed off the U.S. squad by Rogers and Lewis's teammates, who resented Carl's failure to practise with their relay team?

The ranking was more than a matter of pride. Lewis had earned more than 10 times as much as Ben in appearance money and endorsements in 1985. (At Zurich, Lewis's appearance fee was reportedly $25,000, compared to $800 for Ben.) Given the tiny Canadian market, Ben could not begin to catch up until he was ranked first—the prerequisite to international celebrity.

In my view, the two sprinters were hard to separate. Although Ben's best performances of 1985 approached the level of Carl Lewis at *his* best, as in 1983 and 1984, he had yet to match Carl's dominance in the event. But the Lewis of 1985 was clearly sub-par, and I thought that Ben had performed more consistently that year.

While I shared Ben's disappointment when the rankings came out—Lewis first, for the fifth consecutive year, and Ben second—I wasn't surprised. You needed to knock the champ out before you took his belt away. And we hadn't done that—yet.

Rivalry

By the fall of 1985, the Optimists' support team—the people who would help get our athletes to Seoul three years later—was complete. Super Mike had left us the year before for a better deal in Texas. He was replaced by Waldemar Matuszewski, another defector who had been chief of physiotherapy and regeneration at the Polish National Olympic Centre. The first time I saw Waldemar, I worried that he wouldn't be strong enough; at a wiry six-foot-one and 150 pounds, he was built strangely for his line of work. But he was much stronger than he looked, and brought immense skill and authority to the job. Like Super Mike (but unlike amateurs like myself), Waldemar could loosen muscles through massage without making people sore or bruising any tissue. He'd written his Ph.D. thesis on electronic muscle stimulation, a technique used within the Eastern Bloc since the 1950s but still considered novel in the West. Similar in theory to acupuncture, EMS can isolate the tiniest nerve point for a wide range of effects. It can relieve pain, reduce swelling, and increase circulation to the treated muscle, thereby hastening recovery from injury or fatigue. As an adjunct to weightlifting and other strength work, EMS can also improve an athlete's strength and explosive power.

With Waldemar and Dr. Astaphan in place, we were missing just one more player: a professional agent. I'd actively sought one for Ben and Tony the season before, when both were getting less than the going rate for Olympic finalists. Tom Jennings, the agent who represented Desai and Mark, had turned us down. He said that I was the problem—that he preferred to deal with athletes who were running on their own, without coaches. "What's the first thing you're going to do if an athlete is sore or if his performance is sub-par going into a meet?" he asked me.

"I'll pull him out of the competition," I replied.

"Exactly," Jennings said. "I can't have that kind of interference. When I guarantee athletes for a meet, they have to be there."

Jennings was right. There was no way I could defer to his mode of operation; I would never gamble my athletes' future by running them injured. In October 1985, I found an agent who was willing to work with us on my terms: the Virginia-based Larry Heidebrecht, who had recently left the high-powered International Management Group to go with a new company. We had a strong bargaining position with Larry, since a two-year, non-competition clause in his separation agreement with IMG precluded him from representing all the top stars that he'd previously pursued. He would sink or swim with our people; they would not have to vie with more established names for the opportunities that came Larry's way. Because of his restrictions, he was also willing to hunt for meets for our lower-level athletes, where his commissions—10 percent of appearance fees—wouldn't even pay for his phone calls.

As Larry took stock of our affairs, it became clear that our naivety had been costly. In Ben's four-year Adidas contract, which Optimist founder Ross Earl had negotiated as a favour, the company had escaped the standard "roll-over clause," in which 50 percent of an athlete's bonus money for medals and records was added to his or her base fee for the following year. (Adidas would pay Mark McKoy 20 percent *more* than Ben in late 1987, when Ben was already the world champion and world-record holder in the most marketable event.) Larry understood the rules of the game—he wouldn't press meet directors to give Ben financial parity with

Carl Lewis in 1986, even though Ben was now clearly better. He knew that Ben's public image still had some catching up to do. But he also knew how much the market would bear, and all of our athletes benefited.

In the fall of 1985, Dr. Astaphan announced that he had found a new and improved injectable steroid. He referred to it as Estragol (he later identified its generic name as furazabol), and seemed quite excited about its potential. Estragol was similar in molecular structure to Winstrol, the doctor said, but would be gentler on the athlete's system. Astaphan also told me that Estragol would clear the body more reliably than Dianabol. In fact, he asserted that Estragol was virtually detection-proof, since it was one of many steroids the IAAF did not yet test for. (To be on the safe side, we set a minimum clearance time of two weeks.) We put Ben and Tony on a six-week cycle beginning in November, with three shots a week the first three weeks, and two shots a week thereafter. We repeated the cycle the following March for the outdoor season.

Early reviews were mixed. Ben liked Estragol right away—"This is really good stuff," he said—and stacked it for a time with two-milligram Winstrol tablets, which he'd take until he started to feel stiff. Tony preferred Dianabol, but Astaphan refused to let him go back to it. I decided to try the new drug myself to better gauge its effects, and took twice-a-week injections for five weeks. I understood Tony's preference. Unlike Dianabol, Estragol gave me no sense of euphoria or added confidence—there was no emotional kick at all. But I couldn't argue with the results. When I started my cycle, I was bench-pressing barely 200 pounds. Within nine weeks I was up to 360—matching my previous high as an athlete in training 14 years before.

In October 1985, I received a call from the man who would become the most prominent Canadian in track and field after Seoul: Dave Steen, the decathlete. I'd met Steen the previous winter, when the veteran track coach Andy Higgins had asked me to help some of his athletes at the University of Toronto Track Club with their speed work. I'd also assisted Steen's wife, Andrea, when she set a Canadian record for the 400 metres in 1984. Now Steen, citing a personality conflict, told me he could no longer work with Higgins. Would I coach him instead? I called Higgins and tried to effect a reconciliation, but Steen was adamant. He wasn't going back. "Will you help me or not?" he demanded. I agreed to help. For the next three years, I worked with Steen three times a week.

Steen told me he wasn't interested in steroids, and I never pressed him on the point. But he was curious about vitamin B12 and inosine (both of them permitted substances), and for these I referred him to Dr. Astaphan.

As we approached the indoor season, it was evident that Ben was still improving at a linear rate—about six hundredths per year in the 100 metres—at an age when many athletes begin to level off. (He had turned 24 in December 1985.) With any luck at all with the weather, this would be the year that Ben would break the 10-second barrier.

On January 15, 1986, Ben set a world record at an invitational meet in Osaka of 6.50 seconds in the 60 metres. Ben advanced overnight from star to superstar in Japan. He even began to get some serious recognition back in Canada, which had generally overlooked Ben's World Cup triumph in Australia amid the hubbub surrounding the Toronto Blue Jays' drive to a divisional baseball championship. (Ben's indoor record received little notice in the U.S., however, where the media gave more play to Soviet Sergey Bubka's pole vault, the other world mark set at the Japanese meet. Such was the power of Lewis-mania; no other sprinters were perceived to exist.)

Osaka marked the beginning of a dominant indoor season for Ben. He won eight straight indoor sprints, a rare streak for such short and unforgiving races, where a bad start will eliminate even the fastest man. Ben also won Toronto's Maple Leaf Indoor Games—the first Canadian to do so since Harry Jerome prevailed in 1963. By season's end Ben had captured the Grand Prix event championship for the 60 metres, awarded annually to the sprinter with the best record over that demanding circuit.

But all of this was mere prelude to the Bruce Jenner Meet in San Jose that May, when Ben would renew his now-celebrated rivalry with Carl Lewis. (Ben had to face this challenge on his own; there was no money in our budget for me to accompany him.) Portrayed by the local media as an ornery Canadian who begrudged Lewis the number-one ranking, Ben shot to the lead and was never threatened, winning in 10.01. Lewis, hampered by a false start and possibly by knee problems, ran second in 10.18, a world behind.

Early that summer, after Ben won the Canadian National Championships in 10.07, a race disrupted by several false starts, Lewis won *his* national championships in a wind-aided 9.91. Carl immediately began boasting that he would destroy Ben—he would "kick his ass," to be precise—at Ted Turner's Goodwill Games in Moscow that July. Lewis claimed he hadn't properly prepared for the Jenner meet—an alibi I found especially grating, since Ben lost to Lewis in Modesto even earlier the year before and had never used the calendar as an excuse. The Goodwill Games, Carl insisted, would tell the true story.

I was not concerned; judging from the other times at the U.S. nationals, I equated Lewis's performance to a 10.01 or higher, and felt confident that Ben was still ahead of him. I became less comfortable in Moscow, however, after Ben's starting blocks slipped as he false-started. (The slip—in which the blocks' aluminum spikes actually pierced and clawed through the track surface—was caused by a warped set of blocks, a worn track, and the extreme force generated by Ben's start. He'd asked for new blocks before the race, but the Soviet official on hand didn't speak English.)

Now Ben faced a double-whammy. Not only would his reaction be inhibited by the false start, but he'd have to modify his position and drive out less explosively to make sure his blocks stayed in place.

As I'd feared, Ben failed to get clear early, and Lee McRae, the quick-starting American indoor champion, stayed ahead to the 60-metre point. But Ben blew past him with that middle surge I'd come to count on, and crossed the line in 9.95 seconds. It was the fastest time ever run at sea-level, two hundredths faster than Lewis's best legal time, and just two hundredths off Calvin Smith's altitude-boosted record—a record that Ben probably would have broken with a normal start. We now knew he was ready to go as low as 9.90, given the right conditions. Ben had outpaced our projections yet again.

Nigeria's Chidi Imoh finished second in 10.04. Lewis, who'd never been within hailing distance of the lead, ran third in 10.06. The balance of power between Ben and Carl had irrevocably shifted, a fact that the gathered media in Moscow were slow to grasp. Only one reporter cornered Ben for an interview immediately after the race; all the rest trailed a sullen Lewis off the track and into the locker room. If they were looking for provocative quotes, they got them. The meet had been too soon after the U.S. nationals, Carl complained. Inflated by his nascent recording career, which he promoted by singing the U.S. national anthem at various meets, Lewis asserted that he was too "multi-faceted" to focus solely on running. (A Lewis single bombed in the U.S. but sold well in Sweden.) He refused to attend the Goodwill medal ceremony and left the track with a put-down for Ben: "This seems to be really important to him. Me? I'm just biding my time." Taking up Carl's cause after the race, a gullible reporter pointed to Lewis's outside interests and asked Ben what *he* did away from the track. Angered by the irrelevant question, Ben shot back that he watched "Roadrunner" cartoons. Nobody got the joke.

In early June, a few hours before the Harry Jerome Meet got underway in Vancouver, I had lunch with Chuck DeBus. When I mentioned that the meet would be drug-tested, he stared at me in panic. "Why didn't anyone tell me?" he moaned. "I wasn't planning to have my people tested until our nationals." (The TAC Outdoor Championships were scheduled for two weeks later.)

Since only a few tests were planned, DeBus kept his group in the meet with the hope that no one would be caught. But one of his female athletes was selected for testing—a frightening development, since she'd been taking 10 milligrams of Dianabol and another 10 milligrams of Anavar daily up to that very morning.

DeBus directed her to drink a pint of vinegar in a last-ditch effort to mask the steroids, a ploy of unproven reliability. In any event, the woman tested negative.

It appeared that DeBus wasn't the only American to be caught by surprise in Vancouver. Several top American pole vaulters missed at low heights, allowing them to leave the stadium before they could be collared for a test.

The cold war between Ben Johnson and Carl Lewis was now fodder for headlines. It hadn't always been that way. Early on in our encounters, Carl was quite friendly toward me and the rest of our group. For all of his style excesses—the pointed white-rimmed glasses, the orange-and-black Harlequin tights, the Grace Jones flat-top—I couldn't help but like him, and I was charmed by his parents, whom I'd met on the circuit in 1982.

That same year, I ran into Lewis at Zurich just after he'd competed at the USOC Sports Festival in Indianapolis. Had it not been for a dubious foot foul, he would have broken Bob Beamon's 14-year-old world record in the long jump with a fantastic leap of more than 30 feet. As we chatted in our hotel's game room, Carl said he couldn't believe he'd left the U.S. without the record. When I suggested that he might get it in Zurich, or at the next meet, Lewis was strangely pessimistic: "No, it's all downhill from here."

Unlike some other people, I never minded Lewis's bowing and waving after he'd won a race. When Carl and Edwin Moses— the two biggest stars in track at the time—feuded over this issue, I thought Lewis was on the mark when he noted that he wasn't performing brain surgery. Sometimes we forget that sports is a show—that the athletes are out there to entertain. (In this respect Carl followed the colourful Charlie Greene, the brilliant 100-metre man of the late 1960s. When asked why he always raced in sunglasses, Greene peered at the reporter and breathed, "Re-entry, man.")

Lewis seemed to change in 1983, when his performances—and financial rewards—left the rest of the track world behind. Lewis felt—not unjustifiably—that everyone was pitted against him. He stopped associating with other athletes, and his posturing became more adversarial—after all, who were *they* to talk about *him*? After winning his three gold medals at Helsinki, he declared, "I am Carl Lewis, of the United States of America, and there is only one person I answer to—the Lord."

By 1984, as the Olympics approached and he appeared on the cover of *Time* twice in three weeks, Carl seemed to lose all perspective. "There are going to be some absolutely unheard-of things coming from me," he predicted. Meanwhile his manager, the diminutive Joe Douglas, bragged that Lewis would become a bigger star than singer Michael Jackson. All over the globe, meet directors cringed as Douglas pressed for first-class plane tickets, limousines, and lavish hotel suites. (As Andreas Brügger, the Zurich meet director, once told me, "It was so nice to have your group here. Douglas and his demands make me want to vomit.")

From a marketing standpoint, the Los Angeles Olympics proved to be Lewis's glory and his downfall at the same time. He'd accomplished everything he'd set out to do: swept his four golds, matched Jesse Owens. But all the living-colour exposure was double-edged. People didn't like Lewis any more than before; if anything, they liked him less. They found him aloof when he stayed in posh lodgings outside the Olympic Village; too rehearsed when he carried a gigantic American flag around the track; less than heroic when he passed on four chances to break Beamon's long-jump record, thereby saving energy for the 200 metres and the relay—and his cherished four-medal sweep.

I thought Carl had been wrongly maligned. His decision to move outside the Village was perfectly sensible, given the miserable state of accommodations there. (Ben would make the same choice in 1988, to no audible outcry.) And Lewis acted with proper self-concern in the long jump. The public didn't know that he was protecting a slight hamstring strain; he hadn't publicized the injury, out of concern that his opponents would try to aggravate it by pushing him harder in the heats. The journalists probably wouldn't have attacked Lewis so fiercely if he hadn't disappointed them with a pre-recorded message—rather than a personal appearance for interviews—after his victory in the 100 metres. In any case, a swirling wind on the day of the long-jump finals made a world record highly unlikely.

(The record notwithstanding, Lewis had already proven to knowledgeable observers that he was the greatest long jumper in history, and far superior to Bob Beamon. Beamon's record of 29 feet, 2-1/2 inches, set at the 1968 Olympics in Mexico City, has long been held up as one of the premier feats in the history of sport. In fact, it was a solid but unremarkable effort. Like the 1968 Olympic sprinters, several of whom also set world records, Beamon was aided by Mexico City's thinner air. In addition, he benefited from a gusting tailwind which seemed to far exceed the international limit of two metres per second—about 4.5 miles per hour—beyond which a record is negated. Lynn Davies, the British gold medallist in the event in 1964, later told me that both he and the American Charlie Mays had exceeded 28 feet in their warm-ups, just before Beamon's historic leap—well past the previous world record of 27 feet, 4-3/4 inches—and could barely wait to take their official turns. But Beamon got one more huge break: He jumped fourth, ahead of his top competitors. The first three jumpers fouled. Beamon landed beyond the optical sighting device, and by the time officials had measured the jump manually, the tailwind had died and a late after-noon rain had begun to fall. Devastated, the other finalists failed to break 27 feet. Beamon himself never jumped as far as 28 feet after that day.)

"We're on the frontier," Joe Douglas had announced going into the Games. "We want Carl to be identified with one major company, the way O.J. Simpson is with Hertz or Bob Hope is with Texaco." But the marketers picked up on the public's disaffection, and Lewis failed to land a single major ad campaign despite his four medals. While Mary Lou Retton beamed her way to riches with Wheaties and McDonald's, Carl was left out in the corporate cold. It probably didn't help when Douglas claimed that his client had rejected $100,000 for a single track meet, and would not sign with the National Football League (for which Lewis had no known interest) for less than $1 million a year.

Our relationship with Lewis didn't really sour until 1985, when Ben beat him for the first time at Zurich. Carl insisted at the time that he was coasting after Los Angeles. He voiced similar sentiments after losing to Ben in San Jose and Moscow in 1986, and the pattern was set. Carl had always been number one, and he couldn't adjust—especially since he knew that the difference between number one and number two in the 100 metres meant several millions of dollars a year.

Number One

In July 1986, we had scheduled a tune-up meet for about half of our national team in Birmingham. The rest of the team, which totalled well over a hundred people, planned to travel on ahead to Edinburgh and settle in early for the Commonwealth Games, to begin a week later. We were about to depart from London when Gerard Mach got the bad news: the Commonwealth Games Association of Canada would not pay to house any of our athletes before the meet officially began, which meant we had about 50 extra people to put up in Birmingham. At a rest stop en route, I found Gerard brooding in the back of the bus. I asked him if he'd called Andy Norman, the British Amateur Athletic Association (AAA) official in charge of the meet, about our need for additional lodgings.

He looked at me dolefully. "I can't call Andy," he said. "I haven't got a cent, we've spent it all—I don't have enough for lunch today. What if Andy turns us away—what if he says that he only wants five or six stars? We're just going to land on his doorstep and pray that he takes us all in."

At that point I grew even more worried than Gerard. I had first encountered Andy Norman seven years before, at the tri-meet in

Gateshead with Britain and Kenya. My job at that time was to assist our team's head coach, John Redmond, an amiable high school principal and a Catholic priest. (To avoid making people uncomfortable, Father John rarely wore a clerical collar.) On the night before our competition, Norman came steaming toward us in the hotel lobby. With his dishevelled hair, a pot belly that peeked through an unbuttoned shirt, and lowslung pants barely clinging to his hips, he looked like a cross between Andy Capp and Long John Silver, with an attitude to match.

"All right, who's in charge of this bloody team here?" he snapped.

"I am," said Father John.

"And what's your name then?" Norman barked.

"John Redmond," my head coach replied.

"Then tell me, John, where are your goddamned throwers? What kind of bloody meet do you think this is?" Nobody asked me, but I knew what the problem was: Two of Canada's top throwers had ducked the meet because they knew it would be tested, and they wanted to stay on their steroids as close as possible to the Pan Am Games eight weeks later. I stood beside Father John, cringing.

"Who the hell are my people supposed to throw against?" Norman demanded.

"I don't know," Father John said mildly.

"Well," Norman said, "you get on the bloody phone and tell those bastards back at the CTFA to get some throwers out here!" After expounding at length upon the parentage of said CTFA officials, he stormed off.

For years afterwards I considered Norman a man to be avoided, until his name came up in a conversation I had with Hasely Crawford, the Trinidadian who had won the 100 metres at the 1976 Olympics. "No, you've got him all wrong," Hasely told me. "He's a good man." In Birmingham, after we'd anxiously signed our entire team into the hotel register, Norman proved Hasely right—that his gruffness was a façade. As soon as Cerard explained our plight, Norman agreed to pay for all of the rooms. He even volunteered to arrange for a recreational tour bus for our group. Then Gerard decided to push our luck a bit: "Some of our people would like to be paid for running."

"Oh, yeah?" Norman said. "Let's not beat around the bush. Charlie, I want Ben—how much?"

With nothing to lose (it didn't really matter if Ben ran in the meet or not), I plucked a figure out of the air: "Ten thousand dollars." It was far more than Ben had ever gotten on the circuit.

"No way!" Norman responded, and we went on to negotiate lesser deals for Angella and some of the others. But I thought I'd give Norman one more chance on Ben, and fell in behind him at the hotel's salad bar. We stood silently for a time as we piled up our salads, and finally Norman looked over his shoulder at me and muttered: "Eight." I snapped it up; eight thousand would still be a new high.

I was feeling quite proud of myself when I told Angella that Ben would be running after all. "I know," she said. "I just heard it on the radio." In true rogue's fashion, Norman had the last laugh. If I'd known he'd already publicized Ben's appearance, I could have held firm for the full ten thousand.

The more I saw of the vaunted British track "system," the more I came to realize that Andy Norman was its linchpin. In reality, the British had no system. The AAA was just as chaotic as the CTFA. British coaches were no more competent than those in Canada. Their athletes were successful because Andy had engineered a lucrative revenue-sharing contract with British television. (Many sponsors had turned to track and field after a series of stadium riots scared them away from soccer.) With substantial monetary incentives in place, a sprinter like Linford Christie could quit his day job and begin training full time in 1986. He was able to take the plunge because Norman's contractual coup rewarded British athletes on a preferential basis. (Although Ben was beating Christie consistently in 1986, Christie would be paid 50 percent more at meets within the United Kingdom. In Canada, by contrast, most meets would pay Canadian athletes *less* than they would get anywhere else.) Freed from distractions, Christie made huge strides that year. He went from unranked to fourth in the world in the 100, won the European championship, and confirmed my axiom: You don't get full-time results out of part-time athletes.

It was bitterly cold at the Commonwealth Games, but my athletes overcame the conditions to take 11 medals. Angella staged a comeback after giving birth to a daughter and won a gold in the 200, a bronze in the 100, and a silver in the sprint relay. She had resumed training the previous December but hadn't gone back on steroids until April, when she'd stopped breast-feeding. She travelled with her baby and more than 100 pounds of pre-mixed infant formula. After a meet that summer in Germany I'd lugged the formula through Checkpoint Charlie, the border crossing from East to West Berlin, at the risk of hæmorrhage.

In 1978, Ben hadn't made our Commonwealth Games team. At the 1982 Games, he'd run second in the 100 to Allan Wells. This time around, Ben completed the circle. He won the gold in the 100 in 10.07, tying his own British-soil record, and added another gold in the 4x100 relay and a bronze in the 200. The triple duty in Edinburgh tired him and it showed immediately after the Commonwealth Games in Gateshead, where Ben finished fourth in a sluggish 10.53, his first outdoor loss of the year. When the news got out, Lewis arranged to run in Zurich in August, trumpeting that this race would tell who was best. He joined an imposing field: Chidi Imoh, Calvin Smith, Linford Christie, Harvey Glance, Kirk Baptiste, Marian Woronin. No one was missing. We could hear the drums beating: *Ben's weak; let's get him.*

I felt torn. I wanted Ben to run in Zurich and establish his supremacy, once and for all, but I didn't want to risk losing a near-certain number-one ranking if he were off form. "If you don't feel good," I told him the day before the meet, "you can run the 200 and skip the 100." But Ben insisted that he felt fine, and on race day he appeared ready to do battle. "I talked to my mom this morning and she prayed for me," he said.

For all its build-up, the race was no contest. Ben got a mediocre start, and Lewis was less than three feet behind after 50 metres, well within striking distance. But once again Ben surged, and by

80 metres he had stretched his lead to 10 feet—and then he put on the brakes, raised his right arm (in a show of dominance that would foreshadow Seoul), and almost walked across the line. He finished in 10.03—into an 0.7-metre headwind. The race for second was won by Imoh in 10.23, with Lewis third at 10.25. (I learned later that Carl had been bothered by calcium deposits on his left knee, and required arthroscopic surgery after the season.) Ben had now beaten Lewis three straight times; the vote for number one would be a formality.

A full year before his glory in Rome, I knew that Ben was ready to run in the 9.80s. His grandstanding in Zurich had cost him at least a tenth of a second. His sub-optimal start and the headwind may have cost him another one. After the race, Wolfgang Meier ran down to the track to congratulate me. "He gave away a world record!" the East German coach declared. "If he were my athlete, I'd *strangle* him."

Ben's speed came in handy in his perpetually crowded social life as well. A master of the broken promise and forgotten obligation, he was always in trouble with the women he dated. On some days two or three of them would come out to the track at York University to wait for Ben while he trained. On more than one of these occasions I saw him end practice by hopping a fence, running to his car, and roaring off to avoid an awkward scene.

For a time Ben was going out with one of his Optimist team-mates, a woman with little patience for his shenanigans and farfetched excuses. One evening, according to the gossip, Ben spent a romantic evening with this woman, then left her for a late-night rendezvous with someone else. At the following day's practice, Ben's teammate would have nothing to do with him.

"But *you're* the only one for me, baby," Ben pleaded, in his heavy Jamaican lilt. "I don't care about her."

At that the teammate glared at the nearby parking lot and said, "Ben, that would be a lot more believable if she wasn't sitting in your car right now."

"No, no," Ben insisted, "that's my *cousin*."

In a distressing sidebar to an otherwise stellar season, I learned that Rob Gray, a top Canadian discus thrower and long-time friend, had tested positive for Deca-Durabolin at our national championships and (along with shot-putters Peter Dajia and Mike Spiritoso) would be suspended for 18 months. I had met Rob in 1978, when he was stalled in the 58-metre range. In 1984 he got serious about the sport. He found a full-time coach, asked to train with me for speed work (which offers power benefits to throwers), and went to Dr. Astaphan for a new drug program. Rob was always outspoken about the realities of steroids in his event and had never been discreet about his own use. "I don't see why he needs it," Gerard once told me, before Rob had come to us. "I had an athlete in Poland in 1959, and he was close to number one in the world, and he never took drugs."

But Gerard didn't understand how times had changed. In the late 1950s, a discus thrower could work like a dog—without drugs—and become a top contender with throws of 59 metres. But by 1983, the Canadian Olympic Association had set a *qualifying* standard of 64.50 metres. A thrower could put in his six or eight hours a day, but without steroids he'd have little chance of getting into the Olympics, much less of winning a medal—and what was the point of that?

In April 1984, Gerard phoned me to say he had heard "some stupid rumour" that Rob had thrown 63 metres. I told him he had been misinformed—that Rob had actually thrown 67.32 metres (more than 220 feet), a new Commonwealth record.

I was surprised to hear of Rob's positive test, since Astaphan advised all of his patients against using Deca and Rob had told him he'd never taken it on his own. Astaphan wondered whether the Deca metabolite might be a "rebound" product from other steroids—whether it might, in fact, have been produced by Gray's system. But Rob's appeal on this point was denied, and his athletic career was finished.

Projections

For Ben and myself, 1987 was the year we put it all together—far more gratifying than the Olympic year to follow. After years of revising and refining, I felt confident that my training system enabled my sprinters to perform at their best. In Ben I had a supreme athlete who'd remained free from serious injury. And while Ben's fame was beginning to encroach upon our training, the distractions were still limited and bearable.

We began the season with a two-week fall camp at St. Kitts, Dr. Astaphan's birthplace and Caribbean home. The Sprint Centre's budget had appeared to rule out any camp at all, but Astaphan told us he could get free plane tickets through British West Indies Airlines, and that a local professional association would find housing and cover food costs for the 11 of us at his mother's hotel. (I later found out that Astaphan had paid for our meals himself.)

The island had no track, and weightlifting facilities were primitive, but there were ample compensations. The sprinters ran on a grass field which cushioned their legs. They also trained every morning on the beach in waist-deep water for resistance work. Everyone seemed to be thriving—particularly Ben, who was staying with Dwyer Astaphan, the doctor's younger brother. A local attorney, Dwyer loved a good time and knew where to find it. After Astaphan saw that the duo was out revelling more than the doctor liked, he moved Ben into his mother's hotel. The change of scene failed to slow the two younger men down, however. One evening I entered the hotel lobby to see three young women waiting there unescorted. I watched Dwyer approach them, motion to one, and say, "Ben will see you now." It was audition time—Ben was screening prospective companions upstairs in his room while getting a massage from Waldemar. He settled on a spectacular beauty and squired her around the island for the remainder of the camp. One evening Angella, who was staying down the hall, heard the sounds of passion as she passed Ben's door. "Oh, Ben, you're the best in the whole world," the woman sighed. "Me know, me know," Ben answered in his patois. Here was a man who strived to be number one in every endeavour.

Mazda had signed individual endorsement deals with Ben and Angella the year before, and in the fall of 1986, the company made the rest of my group an offer as well. (As the carmaker was an IMG client, Larry Heidebrecht could not talk to them, and I wound up representing my athletes.) It was agreed that Mazda International and Mazda Canada together would provide individual sponsorships for 14 athletes, to be paid into their trust funds, and would provide club membership dues for our junior athletes. From that point on, our club was known as the Mazda Optimists. Although Ross Earl continued to raise money for our travel costs, he'd surrendered his active role in the operation. Ross had been worn down by the CTFA's ceaseless paperwork and broken promises. He would remain a loyal and supportive friend, but from here on he would root for us from the background.

We'd begun the season's first six-week steroid cycle before breaking for camp: a total of 15 injections of Estragol, stacked with vitamin B12 and inosine. Astaphan stayed in St. Kitts that fall to practise medicine there full time, and I overcame my needle phobia to inject Ben, Tony, and Cheryl Thibedeau at my apartment. (Angella injected herself at home.) Ben was casual about the program and occasionally missed an injection, to no apparent ill effect. He again stacked the Estragol with two-milligram Winstrol tablets, but stopped the latter after ten days when he began to feel stiff.

I was doing what I could to fend off the campaign within the CTFA for random, out-of-competition testing—a policy that I knew would remove Canada from the international picture. In January 1987, I arranged a private, hour-long meeting with Jean-Guy Ouellette, chairman of the CTFA's board of directors, at a hotel near Toronto's airport. Unlike most of the sport's top executives, Ouellette was regarded as a friend to athletes.

While careful to conceal what my own sprinters were doing, I related to Ouellette the facts of life in our sport: how the East Germans and Soviets tested athletes for control purposes *before* their entry into high-level training groups, where steroids were prescribed under tight supervision; how I'd been told that a West German lab pre-tested samples for some of that nation's athletes; how the U.S. had instituted its own non-punitive testing program in 1984.

I was particularly thorough in describing the state of affairs in Great Britain, long the model for Canadian sport and a self-proclaimed paragon of "clean" competition. Although the Amateur Athletic Association. had pioneered "random" testing within Britain in 1986, its program had yet to yield a single positive, and performances there were better than ever. (In April 1988, in a belated stab at credibility, the AAA recorded its first positive random test. The unlucky example was Jeff Gutteridge, a middle-ranked pole vaulter who had already announced plans to retire after Seoul.)

Ouellette seemed shaken by my accounting. He said he would try to verify what I'd told him with meet directors in Europe, and then advise his board of the international situation.

I had shifted from a double- to a triple-periodization schedule, which seemed to keep my athletes fresher. Our first intensive training block would run 12 weeks, from October through December, and culminate in our indoor season. The second block would stretch another eight weeks from March to May, leading to the early out-door events; the third block would consist of five weeks in June and July, and would point toward our national championships, Zurich, and the 1987 World Championships in Rome. The idea was to stair-case our performances to peak at the most important events. Minor meets were selected by the calendar to fit into our training sched-ule; they were less ends in themselves than speed sharpeners for the bigger prizes.

In addition to the ten-day taper periods before major meets, my sprinters would rest for four or five days between training blocks. It was this overall plan—the three periods, the extended recoveries, the incorporation of minor meets into our training program, the limited steroid dosages and durations—that enabled Ben to compete more frequently than any of his international rivals, until he became known around the circuit as "Robocop."

In 1987, Ben would run 44 outdoor races (including heats), more than double the load of the typical East German sprinter. Because the East Germans took larger doses of steroids for longer periods, they gained a greater rebound effect but also peaked in a narrower frame. There would be only a matter of weeks between the end of their clearance time and their inevitable performance crash from steroid withdrawal. That schedule suited their national program, since the G.D.R. focused each year on a few high-prestige meets. But the plan was more complicated for a Western athlete—and especially for a star like Ben, whose appearance fees were now into five figures. My job was to give Ben as many opportunities as possible to make money, yet keep him fresh enough to win when it counted. It was the most delicate of balancing acts, and we would play it perfectly in 1987.

On January 15th of that year, Ben ran a 6.44 in Osaka—six hundredths better than his previous world record for 60 metres. By my calculations, the 6.50 he'd run indoors in 1986 had been equivalent to a record-tying 9.93 in the 100, which he would have attained in Zurich had he run all the way through. A 6.44 pointed squarely to the 9.80s.

Ben passed one milestone after the next that indoor season. At his next stop, in Perth, Australia, he ran a hand-timed (and wind-aided) 9.7 in the 100, the fastest hand time in memory. In Ottawa, on January 31st, both Ben and Angella broke the world records for 50 metres—a first for two sprinters from the same group. Angella's race appeared to put her within range of Ashford's record 10.76, though I knew that calculations on the women's side were less reliable. As female sprinters fell short of the males' maximum speed, their acceleration also levelled off sooner—at 40 to 60 metres for women, versus 50 to 70 metres for men. A greater proportion of a woman's race depended on her speed endurance, which would be difficult to assess until Angella began her 120- and 150-metre speed drills in May.

We had planned our first peak for February 21st, at the Canadian National Indoor Championships in Edmonton. Aided by 2,000 feet of altitude and a fast surface, our results showed we were on target. Angella set a new Canadian record for the 60 metres in 7.13, and Ben recovered from a poor start to tie his world record of 6.44.

Then came the World Indoor Championships in Indianapolis on March 7. In the 60 metres Ben got out first and widened his margin with every stride. He finished in 6.41, yet another record. Ben was moving so fast that he flipped over the waist-high restraining wall 20 metres past the finish line and landed on his back, unhurt, on a concrete floor; like the East Germans in Los Angeles back in 1983, he had outstripped the arena. Ben had met our first-period goal: to set a record on the day when it counted the most.

Angella entered the meet as a distinct underdog against Nelli Cooman, the short-legged Dutch accelerator who had been thrashing the East Germans and everyone else indoors for years, and who held the world record for 60 metres at 7-flat. Angella had upset Cooman in Ottawa, but was still shaky after wrenching her back on a decrepit track in Hamilton before the nationals. The final in Indianapolis was close from the start, but it appeared that Angella had gotten up at the finish line, and she was interviewed as the winner for television. Forty-five minutes after the race, the photo was released, and we found that Cooman had won after all—she had out-leaned Angella and prevailed by an eyelash, by a *thousandth* of a second, in 7.08. Angella was devastated, but I could see a bright side: She was running faster than ever before. If she held form, I thought she might win in Rome in the summer to come.

Ben's new record served to revise my projection of his 100-metre time downward, to between 9.85 and 9.80. Gerard agreed, granting my assumption that Ben would run his last 40 metres as well as he had in Zurich the year before. This was not quite a given; it would be tougher for Ben to maintain his Zurich pace throughout, since his faster starts were now burning more energy out of the blocks. To be conservative, I predicted a 9.85 for Rome, when Ben should be peaking. The Italian sportswriters I spoke to after Indianapolis thought this quite reasonable. Inveterate handicappers themselves, they were all aware that he was headed under 9.90, though how far under remained a matter of debate.

Elsewhere, however, my prediction was doubted and even mocked, particularly in the U.S. press. Frank Dick, director of coaching for the British national team, told the media that Ben was sure to "blow up and die" if he went out at his Indianapolis pace in a 100-metre race. But as the old saying went, time would tell.

Aside from Ben's heroics, the 1987 indoor season was noteworthy for one other development: the introduction of drug testing for indoor meets by The Athletics Congress in the United States. Strange events conspired to keep some elite performers out of the testing rooms. At one meet, a top-ranked sprinter couldn't even make the 60-yard final. A number of pole vaulters, after a banner year in 1986, were now falling short of their previous performances—a pattern which can indicate a cutback in an athlete's steroid protocol. On the Grand Prix circuit in Europe, one star vaulter performed so erratically at drug-tested meets that the directors would no longer offer him an appearance fee—they would pay him only by the centimetre.

To Rome

Our early outdoor season began inauspiciously. At a May meet in Provo, Utah, Ben's calf cramped during the race, leaving him less than a week to recover for the year's first confrontation with Lewis in Seville, Spain. It was a race I'd looked forward to, and the first time that Ben would be paid more to run than Carl, but now we'd be at a disadvantage. There was no guarantee that the spasm—a death blow in a tough contest—would not recur.

Ironically, Joe Douglas had presented us with an out before the mishap. He told Larry Heidebrecht that he hadn't known Ben would be entered in Seville, and that the premature match-up might cost both camps a more lucrative deal later on. Would Larry agree to call the meet promoter and endorse Douglas's proposal to feature Ben in the 100 and Carl in the 200? Larry said it was out of our hands, since we'd known Carl was in when we signed with the promoter, but that if Douglas could do something on his end, it would be fine with us. In the end, despite rumours that Carl would switch to the 200, he squared off against Ben in the 100 as planned.

Fifty metres into the race, though Ben was still four feet ahead, I could tell we were in for a struggle; the cramp had flattened his mid-race surge. But while Lewis came up fast at the end, Ben hung on to nip him at the wire by a hundredth, 10.06 to 10.07. Almost frantic with frustration, Carl carped to the media that he'd been cheated, even after Douglas and I had checked the official photo finish, which clearly showed Ben the winner. Ben had heard enough. "Look, clown," he growled at Lewis, "let's run another one right now—then you'll know who won." The two almost came to blows, and Ben had to be pulled away by his friend Mel Lattany. When asked about the commotion, Ben told the press, "Carl seemed to be confused over who won the race today. Next time I'll make sure he isn't confused."

Lewis didn't let up. Afterwards he told a British magazine that Ben would be "dead meat" in Rome. Carl didn't realize that Ben had been sub-par in Seville. He would have to learn the hard way.

In April 1987, David Jenkins was arrested for his involvement in a Mexican steroid smuggling ring that had brought in $70,000 a week. Jenkins was a many-time British champion and formerly the world's top-ranked 400-metre runner. I'd met him in 1974 during my European tour with Gerard, and found him to be bright and entertaining. His arrest was a major topic of conversation in Seville, since the authorities had looked for Jenkins at a house in San Diego that he'd rented for some famous British athletes.

As Ben's training capacity had increased from season to season, our daily practices—our group had six of them a week, three for speed work and three for slower-tempo running—became more and more intensive. At this point Ben was spending about four hours a day at the track, with a regimen that would have drained a weaker or less well conditioned athlete. On a "speed day" he'd start by jogging a mile, then get a 15-minute massage from Waldemar, followed by 15 minutes of stretching. (He would repeat the stretching after each training segment. Ben was a very loose and flexible athlete, but we weren't about to chance a strain or a pull.) Next came the high-knee-lift exercises: sets of 30-metre runs designed to polish various components of Ben's stride. In these and his other drills Ben's form was now impeccable, and he required few corrections from me, though I occasionally needed to remind him to complete the required number of repetitions. Ben was generally conscientious but no glutton for work, and might do less if left to himself.

After a slow 100-metre run on grass (to continue loosening his muscles), Ben put on his spikes for six runs of 60 metres from a standing start, each a bit faster than the one before. Moving into the blocks, he ran four 30-metre sprints at near maximum while focusing on his starting technique. Then we sharpened his acceleration with our "cone drills," in which Ben would alternate 20-metre sections of hard and easy running.

Finally came the speed drills themselves: runs of 80, 100, 120, and 150 metres, all from a standing start, all at absolute maximum. Everyone ran by themselves at this stage. In part this was to allow me to monitor each of my sprinters but in Ben's case it was also a protective measure for his teammates. He was now so fast at maximum that anyone who tried to stay with him would risk severe injury.

After another stretch and an 80-metre jog, Ben moved on to the weight room. He used two basic lifts: the squat, where he'd start by standing with the weight, then kneel until his quadriceps were parallel to the ground; and the bench press, where he'd lie on his back and lift the bar straight up from the rack. Then he'd move on to pull-downs on the Universal machine, another routine he excelled at; Ben's "lats" (the back muscles under his armpits) had gotten so big that he looked like Rocky the Flying Squirrel. He'd conclude the practice with more stretching and a 45-minute massage.

Apart from our 25 hours a week in training, I spent a good deal of time with Ben off the track, more than with any of my sprinters aside from Angella. Once a month or so Ben would decide that I needed some fun—I didn't have much of a social life at the time—and he'd take me out to one of Toronto's trendy music clubs. "Come on, man, you're sitting around too much, let's go," he'd say, and off we went. We never paid a cover—Ben was a full-fledged celebrity in his hometown by now—and rarely were billed for his beers or my Diet Cokes.

I'd never met anyone who loved music as eclectically as Ben did. He carted his portable compact-disc player everywhere he went, and he listened to *everything*, from reggae to Frank Sinatra. Once Desai was going through Ben's kit bag when he came across a disc of love ballads made by one of those crooners who advertise on late-night television. Desai began scoffing, but Ben cut him short: "What's it to you, man? You don't have to listen."

Ben would also drop by my apartment at any hour, often at one or two in the morning—sometimes to get a steroid injection, at other times to raid my refrigerator or just to chat. We wouldn't talk about track; our favourite subjects were women and cars. Ben wasn't the type to routinely share intimacies. Unlike Angella, a person who liked to talk through what was bothering her, Ben was self-contained and utterly assured. He had no need for a mentor's morale-boosting. For all our differences in age and background, Ben and I shared a typical male friendship—and I sometimes felt that he preferred my undemanding company to that of the women who vied for his time. Late one night he came by and made a sandwich, flicked on the television, and killed 45 minutes in my living room. Then, with no special urgency, he said, "Oh, yeah, got to go—I got someone waiting in the car."

After running a 10.02 in Calgary and a 10.07 in Athens in June, Ben returned home for his next block of intensive training, including his last two weeks of steroid injections for the year. In late July, he entered a ten-day taper period to prepare for our national championships, which would mark the start of the season's most critical period. Ben performed there as we had hoped, winning the 100 in 9.98—the fastest time ever on Canadian soil.

After another ten-day recovery period, he ran three remarkable races within a week: a 10.05 in Malmö, Sweden, on August 10th, despite cold conditions and a slow track; a 10-flat into a headwind in Koblenz, West Germany, on August 13th; and a windless 9.95 in Cologne on August 16th, which matched the world sea-level best he'd set in Moscow the year before. (Angella also won in Malmö and Koblenz, and broke the Canadian record in Cologne with a 10.97.)

Ben had evolved into a true champion. He no longer cared if he started in front, because his mid-race was so good that he knew he'd still win—and as a consequence his starts had become more reliable than ever. As the World Championships loomed closer, Ben also became more serious than before, to the point where he swore off sex for the rest of the season: "Man, I'm going to be *mean* by the time I get to Rome."

But even as Ben reeled off brilliant times with near-mechanical consistency, I wasn't allowed to forget that disaster could strike at any time. It almost happened at Cologne, where a horde of more than 100 photographers were jockeying beyond the finish line to get an unimpeded view of the race. The most reckless among them wound up sitting cross-legged in Ben's lane, just 10 metres past the line, or about 20 metres before Ben could possibly stop. He ran into the man with sickening impact, flipped through the air, and crashed flat on his back on the track—a terrifying moment.

I ran to the scene, but neither Waldemar nor I could get through to Ben. He was ringed by photographers who were determined to record the "news" their member had created. I got into a shoving match with one of them, who proceeded to kick me in the groin. As I weighed my next move, a pair of thick, bare arms shoved my antagonist in the chest and sent him flying, ass over lens cap: Ben to the rescue. While I was relieved to find Ben standing unassisted, I feared that all of our meticulous plans might come undone. With their own meet only three days off, the Zurich representatives in Cologne were nearly as anxious as I was. They asked Waldemar to name the equipment he'd need to work on the bruises and scrapes that mottled Ben's back. "Everything will be waiting for you as soon as you get there," they assured us, and it was.

That Zurich meet will always be special to me. Ben, almost fully recovered, ran a 9.97 into a 1.2-metre headwind—an astounding performance and an ideal set-up for his assault on the world record in Rome. Angella also won in 11.03 against the same wind. It was the first time in the meet's storied history that the men's and women's 100 metres had been won by sprinters with the same coach. I thought back to 1978, when I'd had to watch the *Weltklasse* from the standing-room section. This time around, Andreas Brügger escorted me to the in-field after the award ceremonies and introduced me to the crowd, a rare honour.

Ben's first heat at the World Championships was scheduled for August 29th, giving us time for one last ten-day taper to gather and hone his speed. To allow for jet lag, we headed to Rome a week before the meet. During an otherwise uneventful flight out of Berlin, we came across an in-flight magazine which hyped the imminent clash between Ben and Carl with what could have been a Lewis press release:

"It appeared his [Johnson's] greatest task lay not in realizing his obvious sprinting ability, but in overcoming an almost debilitating stutter. It seemed almost symbolic: while Lewis was smooth and polished in every respect, Johnson was struggling and faltering."

I could see Ben simmering as he read. He hadn't needed any more incentive to crush Lewis on the track, but he'd gotten it anyway. As he later told *Sports Illustrated*, "That became part of my race in Rome."

The offending article proved but a foretaste of Lewis's off-track campaign, as he wooed the international media with champagne conferences from the plush Villa Miani, in the hills overlooking the Vatican. He had "never been healthy" when he'd lost to Ben, Lewis claimed. He'd "always intended to be low key" for the two seasons after the Olympics, he explained. Lewis had found his nirvana— an audience that was willing to listen as long as he wanted to talk. With track's other superstars (notably 1,500-metre stars Steve Cram and Saïd Aouita) all ducking one another by entering different events, the 100 metres was *the* story at Rome, the only contest that really mattered, and Carl was the barker who could pitch it. Ben came into Rome with the five fastest times in the world that year, but you'd never have known it from the newsstands. Every magazine in the city seemed to be stamped with Lewis's picture— and his worldview. "Johnson Chasing Credibility," read *The Times* of London headline. "You Can't Do It, Ben," scoffed *l'Equipe*, the huge French sports daily. (The front page of a Rome paper was plastered with photos of Carl's and Ben's heads atop the bodies of Muhammad Ali and Joe Frazier—an apt analogy, I thought.)

It came down to this: After four straight losses to Ben, Carl was sure he would win this time. He had indeed improved his starts. He knew from his training that 9.93 was in the bag—and 9.90 a definite possibility. But he had made one fatal mistake. He had overlooked the fact that Ben had improved as well, and was drawing away from Lewis and everyone else on two legs.

The gap between Carl's perspective and reality was paralleled by the two press conferences I attended before the meet. At the first, packed with European writers, I answered technical questions: "How can an athlete as strong as Ben keep himself supple and flexible?"; "How can Ben compete so often at such a high level?" But the second conference was dominated by American journalists, who had worshipped at the Lewis altar too long to easily convert.

"Do you think that Ben can become number one?"

"He's been number one for two years now," I replied curtly.

"But aren't you and Ben intimidated by the fact that Carl is the Olympic champion?"

"Not at all," I said. "In 1983, in Helsinki, Carl wasn't intimidated by Allan Wells just because Wells won the Olympics in 1980."

"Won't Ben have trouble getting through the three preliminary rounds here?" (As Lewis also excelled at the 200 metres, his speed endurance was considered an advantage in multiple-round competitions.)

"It's just like any invitational meet," I said. "The only difference is that here you'll coast through the heats, and then you'll meet the guys you always run against in the final."

There was more of the same, but it was clear that I'd never convince these people. Only Ben could do that.

Lewis usually ran faster than he needed to in the heats, the better to intimidate the opposition, but in Rome he outdid himself: a meet record 10.05 in his preliminary heat, a 10.03 in his semi-final. His knee was fine, that much was evident. Ben, meanwhile, bolted to a three-metre lead in his semi, then shut down to cruise home in 10.15. "The way Carl was running the heats, he was setting me up," Ben would tell reporters after his triumph. "But the time to do my running was in the final."

Throughout the week, Ben had seemed preternaturally calm and confident, accepting the Romans' mania—even Ben's mother would be mobbed on the streets—without absorbing it. (There were undeniable benefits to all the fuss. One day, Marcello Mastroianni's tailor measured Ben for three complimentary suits, each worth at least $3,000.) I wasn't doing as well. The tension surrounding big meets always played havoc with my health; the night before the Rome final I'd landed in the hospital with an abscessed tooth, and I was still dizzy from antibiotics the next day. I couldn't believe it when I found Ben dozing in the physio's room during the 90-minute break between the semis and the final. *Everything* was on the line for us. The conditions had set up perfectly for Ben's run at the world record: a friendly tailwind of just under a metre, a fast track, and the best competition. And here was the man of the hour, sleeping. I nudged him awake and urged, "You better start warming up. Everyone else is out there."

"It's hot out there," he said, yawning. "It only takes a few minutes to warm up." Then, just before he went out on the track, he found a few words to settle my nerves: "Don't worry. I'm ready."

Ben was so ready that the media-dubbed "race of the century" was as good as over before the runners' first stride. Ben reacted to the gun in a quicksilver .129 seconds; Carl got off in .196. The difference was nearly seven hundredths, an insurmountable margin against a sprinter who had improved his finish as much as Ben had. (Mel Lattany, watching the race in a London pub, had bet $500 on Ben and gotten 2-1 odds. The instant the race started he turned his back to the screen and said, "Pay up, suckers.")

Lewis was more than three feet behind after the first 20 metres, and he was still more than three feet behind at the tape. This time there was no defiant gesture to mar Ben's finish. He was all business, all the way through. Only at the very end did he break his grim mask of focus. As he glanced up at the big screen and saw his winning margin, he broke into a broad grin.

From the stands I peered at the electronic time board, and thought I saw 9.94. *He missed the record again*, I thought, my heart sinking. *How could he have missed it again?* Then I took a second look and realized I'd misread the numbers: It was *9.84*, according to the photo-eye set slightly past the finish line. The official time of 9.83 was announced a few moments later. The world record had been smashed out of sight.

Carl had finished second in 9.93, surpassing his own personal best by four hundredths. While running at sea level, he had tied Calvin Smith's old record set at altitude. At another time that would have been cause for rejoicing in the Lewis camp. But today it only confirmed that Carl was number two—and further removed from number one than ever. As Ben had promised in Seville, Carl no longer had grounds for confusion.

As the crowd of 70,000 stood and roared, I glanced over at Gerard. He was sitting quietly, in tears; it was the high point of his career.

Ben's joy was edged with vindication. For two years, Lewis had entered each race with promises and left with excuses. But Ben had never guaranteed anything he couldn't deliver—as he made clear in a post-race interview with Dwight Stones of NBC.

"You said you'd run 9.85 and you ran 9.83," Stones began.

"Yah," Ben told the live network audience, "I don't talk shit."

The King

Ben's race in Rome changed everything. It dismantled the stereo-types of the world's two top sprinters—that Ben was the best starter and accelerator in the sport, but that Carl had a higher maximum speed and ran "the best concluding 50 metres of all time," as *Sports Illustrated* put it. By this analysis, pushed hard by the Lewis camp, Carl could remain "fastest" even though Ben beat him time after time.

Ben's overall supremacy could not gain public acceptance un-til after he smashed the world record—and until the full scope of what he'd accomplished had been certified by a team of statisticians from Charles University in Prague. Within hours of Ben's record performance, we had access for the first time to a complete statis-tical breakdown of a 100-metre race, including the eight finalists' times at each 10-metre split (after 10 metres, 20 metres, and so on) and their speeds during different segments of the race. That report confirmed my central premise: that maximum speed, not condition-ing or the ability to relax, was the key factor in any short sprint, and the basis for Ben's supremacy.

I had never bought the theory that Lewis had been the best because he decelerated less than his opponents toward the end of the race. I thought he won because he reached a higher top speed. Because of his relatively gentle acceleration at the start, Lewis might still be behind at 50 to 70 metres, where he reached that top speed. But there was no question that he'd been going much faster than the rest at that point, regardless of his place in the race. Over the last 30 metres, that advantage in sheer speed would produce Carl's trademark charge from behind. And toward the end of the race, no matter how much or little Lewis decelerated, he was descending from a higher point than everyone else, which explained how he continued to gain so much ground to the tape. (The Czech statisticians also demonstrated that some sprinters— Carl and Ben included—might actually *accelerate* during the last 20 to 30 metres, an idea that had been heretofore rejected as an optical illusion.)

Judging from the tapes of Ben's victory in Zurich in 1986, I had estimated that he'd achieved a top speed of 12.1 metres per second—Carl Lewis country—after a middling start. In Rome, Ben had once more matched Lewis's maximum speed, but this time after a maximum start. Ben had expanded his energy envelope to unheard-of proportions.

Although Ben's superior reaction time was decisive, the statistics showed that he would have won handily even had he and Lewis reacted equally well to the gun. In the actual *running* of the race, Ben had seized a margin of three hundredths by the 20-metre mark. He expanded that advantage to five hundredths by 50 metres, maintained it there to 80 metres, and finally gave a little back, to return to a final running margin of three hundredths. Put another way, Ben out-started and out-accelerated Carl (and everyone else), then reached the same maximum speed at an earlier point in his race. The formula was simple—and doomed Lewis to second place for the foreseeable future. More than three inches taller than Ben, Carl's lanky body wasn't suited to match his rival's early acceleration; the longer levers of Carl's legs would always slow him early on. Lewis's only hope was to somehow push his own maximum speed *beyond* 12.1 metres per second—a tall order—and to hope that Ben would not do the same.

By August 31st, the day after Ben's great victory, the busiest man in Rome was Larry Heidebrecht. He began working the sponsor tents outside Olympic Stadium at 7:00 A.M. and kept at it until 2:00 the next morning, a pattern he'd repeat for the next five days. *Everyone* now wanted a piece of Ben. Over the next year, Larry would line up enough deals to make Ben a rich man. The agent's masterpiece was a four-year, $2.3-million (U.S.) contract with Diadora sportswear of Italy—about twice as much as Lewis was reportedly getting from *his* sportswear company.

The sponsors knew what they were buying in Ben: the highest-profile persona in sport, *the fastest man in the world*. I saw what this meant first-hand at a meet in Sardinia immediately after Rome. After Ben ran a 10.10 into a strong headwind to crush a weary field, the crowd went wild. Thousands of people streamed out on the field to try to get to Ben. They nearly trampled their own top distance runner, Stefano Mei, and Saïd Aouita, the multiple world-record holder. All lesser suns were in eclipse.

The media paid its homage as well. By year's end Ben had been voted the world's top athlete by the major press associations, including those in the United States, Italy, West Germany, and the Soviet Union. (In Japan, Ben was voted the world's number one *personality*, a poll which included actors and singers as well as sports figures.)

Ben's sudden pre-eminence represented the return of the 100-metre champion to his rightful place as the king of track and field. The world's fastest human had held the throne for decades, from Charlie Paddock through Jesse Owens to Bob Hayes. But in 1968, when the IAAF began to make the transition from hand to electronic timing, it bungled the job. As an electronic clock would start the instant the gun was fired (eliminating a human timer's reaction gap), times would be more than two tenths of a second slower. Rather than adjust for the change by putting the clocks on a delay, as proposed by East Germany, the IAAF let the new and slower times stand. In so doing, they severed the 100 metres' link to its past progression of world records dating from 1896. They had, in effect, created a new event.

At the 1968 Olympics, the change's impact was masked by Mexico City's altitude, where the benefit of thinner air partially neutralized the change in timing. When Jim Hines won the 100 metres in an electronic time of 9.95, it appeared to be comparable to his hand-timed world record of 9.9 at sea level, though in fact he'd run much faster. (Had Hines been hand-timed in Mexico, he would have recorded a 9.7.) But when Valery Borzov won in 1972 with a 10.14 at sea level (after running a 10.07 in a heat), and Hasely Crawford followed with a 10.06 in 1976, the world's fastest human seemed to be in regression. With no one able to break the 10-second barrier, much less to set a new record, the public wrongly concluded that the sprinters of the day just weren't as good as the people who'd run in the late 1960s. The fans turned their attention to the sport's new kings, milers Sebastian Coe and Steve Ovett, who would break *their* world record five times between 1979 and 1981, racking up record appearance fees along the way.

Hines's world record would stand for 15 years, until 1983, when Calvin Smith ran his 9.93 at similar altitude in Colorado Springs. But Calvin could never repeat his feat at sea level. (Colorado Springs' 7,000 feet of altitude improved 100-metre times by about a tenth of a second.) Moreover, Calvin was a quiet man: it would take a more outsized personality to restore the 100 metres to its place of pride. Enter Carl Lewis—and a new era for the sprints. It wasn't just that Lewis was good. It was that he *knew* he was good—and made the rest of us know it, too. Well-spoken and mediagenic, Lewis brought a talent for public relations that the 100 metres sorely needed—and found a U.S. media machine hungry for a homegrown megastar. (As *Time* magazine enthused: "Gentler than a superman, more delicate than the common perception of a strong man, Lewis is physically the most advanced human being in the world…. How fast he runs, how far he jumps, may serve to establish the precise lengths to which men can go.") It didn't seem to matter that Carl had never held an individual world record. Like Muhammad Ali, he was simply, indubitably, the greatest.

Carl paved the way for us. His post-L.A. persona as painted by the press—vain, arrogant, self-righteous—made Ben seem doubly modest and unaffected. Where Carl would brag endlessly about what he was going to do, Ben let his legs do the talking.

Lewis also blazed a trail with the meet directors. By 1984, Carl was refusing to run preliminary heats on the Grand Prix circuit, demanding a bye into the finals. The directors grumbled at this high-handedness (and at its impact on their box office), but gave in to it—and once they did, they ultimately had to extend the same courtesy to Ben. By running fewer heats, Ben could compete in more meets with less fatigue. I agreed with Joe Douglas when he said, "Why run twice to get paid once when you can run twice and get paid twice?"

Most of all, Lewis created excitement. His presence—and pre-race hype—defined an event as important. It mattered because Carl was there, and that was that. When Ben became a star in 1986, it wasn't because he broke the world record for 60 metres, or because he won in Zurich, or even because he ranked number one at year's end. Ben broke through because he was *the man who beat Carl Lewis*. Carl certified Ben's greatness to the public, not to mention the commercial sponsors. Lewis's magnificence was beyond dispute. How magnificent, then, must be the man who could defeat him?

Three days after losing the 100 in Rome, Lewis dropped a bombshell over British television. "There are gold medallists in this [Rome] meet who are definitely on drugs," he said, in a statement seized upon by the world press. "That race [the 100] will be looked at for many years, for more reasons than one.... I don't think it's fair to point fingers. I'm not bitter or anything at anyone. But there's a problem and I just want to take a stand.... If I were to jump to drugs, I could do a 9.8 right away." (Later on, Joe Douglas would insist to me that Lewis had been misquoted—a claim refuted by the videotape.)

Though stung by Carl's words, Ben addressed his foe's behaviour calmly to the press. "When Carl Lewis was winning everything, I never said a word against him—he won and that was it," Ben said. "And when the next guy comes along and beats me, I won't complain about that, either."

Come-down

I used to think the coaching life would get easier once I had a big star—that I wouldn't have to scratch for funding and coax meet directors into entering my lesser runners. I thought my efforts and athletes would finally get the respect they deserved—even at home in Canada, a nation uncomfortable with success.

In the fall of 1987, I found out how wrong I'd been. Ben's new status brought new problems—bigger problems. And while the pressures were greater than ever, I would get even less support than before.

According to *The Toronto Sun*, our Mazda Optimist group—and its high-profile performances—would lure more than $1.1 million in corporate sponsorship revenues to the CTFA over the coming season, or about three times the association's competitive budget just three years earlier. (After commissioning a painting of Ben in a national team uniform, for example, the CTFA marketed thousands of posters and kept 85 percent of the proceeds.) Sport Canada also prospered from Ben's fame—and from our politicians' fevered expectations for the coming Olympics. By 1988, the agency's empire building had progressed until 900 employees were on hand to service only 832 carded athletes. (Although Sport Canada was also technically responsible for serving the masses of developing and recreational athletes, grass-roots sport was actually administered by volunteers in the provinces.)

Sport Canada would provide staff to the CTFA, but without any input from below as to what was needed; all of its offers were strictly take it or leave it. Although the CTFA now had 21 employees, many in esoteric roles, Gerard and his daughter were left alone to work until 3:00 in the morning on travel arrangements for the team.

Insulated from reality, a Sport Canada task force issued *Towards 2000*—a more moderate fantasy than the CTFA's *Project 2000* of 1984, but fantasy nonetheless. Strongly endorsed by Otto Jelinek, then minister for fitness and amateur sport, the report expressed a determination "to enable athletes with talent and dedication to win at the highest level of international competition." To that end, Canada would be expected to:

* Place among the three leading Western nations (with the U.S. and West Germany) and rank among the top six to eight nations overall at the 1992 Olympics in Barcelona.

* Place among the top six nations at the 1992 Winter Olympics in Albertville, France.

* Win medals in 18 of 28 Summer Olympic sports and in 6 of 10 Winter Olympic sports in 1992.

* Place first in the 1990 Commonwealth Games. (Canada would actually finish a weak third behind England and Australia.)

Such lofty goals would have pushed our national teams to the limit, even with a massive infusion of money and a state-supported doping program. But the Sport Canada braintrust never provided the funds, nor would it admit to the worldwide realities of steroid use. While Sport Canada freely took bows for our achievements, it failed to match the resolve of its foreign counterparts in providing non-punitive testing programs. Like the First World War generals who dined on pâté while their troops were slaughtered like live-stock, our diffident bureaucrats lacked the will to win the war they'd declared.

From the trenches, where I stood, the 1988 season looked grim. We had no money for warm-weather training camps in this, an Olympic year. (I eventually hustled two expense-paid training camps and two competitive tours in Europe for my group.) Our organization was still held together with chicken wire and spit. But in the wake of Ben's world record, there was more at stake now, and more resentment—both within and outside our group. Rather than build upon our success with more funding, the CTFA was cutting us off. Even as it milked Ben as a cash cow, the officials proposed to withdraw his carding subsidy and travel allowance (a total of $9,800 a year), reasoning that he no longer needed the assistance. I persuaded them that such a move would create more ill will on Ben's part than it could possibly be worth.

I was now expected to raise money to pay for our Sprint Centre personnel, allowing the CTFA to redirect its resources elsewhere. Upon returning from Europe one day, I discovered that the association had fired my assistant coach and the centre administrator—two-thirds of my staff. (The CTFA apparently failed to grasp that the Mazda sponsorship money went directly to my athletes, and was not available to support the Sprint Centre.) Dr. Astaphan had never been paid and was tired of waiting. Waldemar wanted a raise. Everyone felt overworked and under-appreciated, and I couldn't blame them.

I felt overwhelmed by it all, from the daily grind of planning work-outs for 20 athletes (including Desai and Mark, who rejoined our group in October) to the morale problems and in-house squabbling. Chronically exhausted by the stress and long hours, I nearly quit that fall, after my father died. There seemed nothing left in coaching for me. I had reached the apex in Rome; all else would be anti-climax, including the Olympics. If Ben won the gold at Seoul, he would merely be doing the expected. If he lost, he and I would be monumental failures.

A large part of the pressure came from Ben himself. Bowing to outside obligations, he resumed training three weeks late that fall, missing half of his initial steroid cycle. I had to juggle his practices around outside obligations which had him jetting away several times a month, often on long hauls. In contrast to our charmed existence of 1987, when everything went according to plan, 1988 would be a year for cutting corners and hoping for the best.

Ben's appeal was particularly strong in star-crazy Japan, where he'd emerged as an international figure with his world indoor records in Osaka in 1986 and 1987. The Japanese adopted Ben as their own. They brought to the relationship a concentrated population, a vast domestic market, and a favourable exchange rate. (The Japanese paid Ben in U.S. dollars, which made everyone happy; while the U.S. dollar was weak against the yen, the Canadian dollar was weaker still.) By that winter Larry Heidebrecht had negotiated a wide range of deals there, from VISA Japan to Urbanet, a large commercial developer. Kyodo, a gas and oil company, ran a contest to give away 10,000 Ben Johnson jackets—and reportedly got two million entries. The company also featured Ben in a television commercial, which aired thousands of times in the months before the Olympics. Over the last six years, Ben had made the 28-hour round-trip flight to Japan 29 times, 20 of them strictly for business and 9 for competitions.

As far as I was concerned, Ben had earned his new prosperity. He'd paid his dues with years of dedicated work in near-poverty, and if he wanted a house in the suburbs for his family or a Ferrari Testarossa to tool around in, more power to him. But superstars aren't like the rest of us, and I couldn't help but be disturbed by some of the changes in Ben. He saw so much money being thrown his way that he lost all sense of proportion. One day he called me for advice about an offer from a supermarket chain to cut a ribbon at a new store in Toronto. Ben wasn't sure the fee was high enough.

"How much are they paying you?" I asked.

"Sixty thousand dollars."

"For cutting a *ribbon*?" I couldn't believe it. "If I were you," I told him, "I'd take the money and run like hell before they change their minds."

As the world's number one, Ben now expected to be catered to. He voiced resentment over having to share me with other athletes, especially the younger ones who'd accompanied us on tour. I had to remind him that he didn't pay my salary. At one point Ben asked me to oversee his work-outs in the morning, apart from everyone else's. I declined; I was already putting in 70 hours a week, and had no desire to push it to 90. But Ben got his way that March, when he refused to join the rest of the Mazda group at our training camp in Guadeloupe. It was too boring there, Ben complained; there was no English-language TV. I was forced to stay in Toronto to make sure Ben trained properly, thereby missing time with my other athletes.

There were times, too, when Ben surprised me with his need for my approval. At the *Toronto Sun* Indoor Games in January 1988, where Ben broke the world record for 50 yards, Angella tied the world record on the women's side. It was an important day for her; after running miserably in several previous indoor meets, she was finally beginning to return to her 1987 form. Angella was giving interviews to a few people when Ben entered the press area. The reporters flocked to him, leaving Angella in mid-sentence. I'd already congratulated Ben after the race, and I had what seemed a simple choice: Should I offer encouragement to the deserted Angella or join the scrum around Ben? I chose Angella, and never thought twice about it—until I heard from Larry that Ben was upset that I'd ignored him.

Perhaps it was Ben's need for my affirmation that made me stay on—that for all the adulation Ben received from his fans and his sponsors, there remained something fundamentally important about the coach-athlete bond. As much as I might have wished otherwise, our work together was not yet complete. World records would always be broken, but a victory in Seoul would be something else—something to last. As Ben put it, "The gold medal is something people remember. It is something no one can ever take away from you."

As I prepared my athletes for the Olympics, I continued to fight a rear-guard action against the random-testing zealots within the CTFA. The association ultimately approved random testing in December, but no tests were implemented until after Seoul.

Meanwhile, with Dr. Astaphan still in St. Kitts, I was running short on supplies. I bartered two bottles of our injectable B12-inosine mixture to Dave Steen in exchange for 100 hypodermic needles, more than enough to last our group for one six-week steroid cycle.

After beginning his winter season in fine form in Canada, Ben travelled to Europe with the rest of our team in February for a series of five indoor meets. He won the 60 metres in Madrid in 6.48, then went on to Sindelfingen, West Germany. There Ben *jogged* through his heat in a dazzling 6.46, the surest sign we'd had so far that he was on track to break his world record in Seoul. In the final Ben pulled away to a huge margin—and then, 20 metres from the finish, he broke stride and limped through the tape in 6.50. He'd strained his hamstring, and the remainder of his indoor season would have to be cancelled. His training toward the most important race of his life would be suspended for at least two weeks.

It was Ben's first injury since 1984, and a good deal of hindsight was expended on where we'd gone wrong. It was easy to blame the business deals which had disrupted Ben's fall training schedule, but I faulted myself as well. In both Madrid and Sindelfingen I'd given in to the meet directors' pressure for Ben to run in the 60-metre heats as well as the finals. The Madrid runs were probably most costly, as the short straightaway there had forced Ben to jam on his brakes—twice—to keep from crashing into a wall. As I watched Waldemar set to work on Ben, I thought back to a meet in Cologne in 1982, where Carl Lewis's father kept repeating, "I don't like those heats." Sure enough, Carl had proceeded to pull a muscle in the final there.

Then again, Ben may have been lucky to avoid injury as long as he did, even with the best training and massage. World-class sprinters are like exotic sports cars: superb in performance, but constantly in need of servicing and subject to breakdown. While coaches and physios do their best to prepare their athletes for the violent forces of sprinting, there are times when the strain is too much.

Our first priority with Ben was to reduce his leg's swelling, so as to speed the healing process by restoring the flow of nutrients to the wound. To receive Waldemar's three treatments a day, Ben stayed with us through the remainder of the European series. He was such a big draw that he was paid 50 percent more *not* to run—to simply show up and help promote the meets—than any other athlete had ever received to compete indoors. But Ben's stardom also set back his recovery. Two days after the injury, he agreed to a media photo session in Karlsruhe. Something got lost in the translation, and word leaked out that Ben would be signing autographs. Suddenly we were swarmed by hundreds of shouting kids. They came over the in-field wall and were on us like army ants, knocking Ben to the ground and piling on. By the time we escaped, Ben had been kicked in his bad leg, causing the torn muscle to bleed again. It cost us at least another week of training.

I had always thought that Carl Lewis's security precautions were part of his celebrity routine. But now I saw that Carl knew how to play this game, while we were still novices. Our baptism had come after the World Championship race in Rome, when an ABC television representative asked for a meeting with us in the stadium to plan future events. Ben didn't show, and finally the Canadian team manager came to explain that the police had prevented Ben from entering the stands. He'd become a safety hazard. If the public saw Ben, they'd stampede to get to him—someone might be killed.

By the time we reached Genoa, the stop after Karlsruhe, Ben had resolved to be more cautious with his adoring fans. After slipping into a changing room inside the stadium, he discovered that hundreds of people were lying in ambush outside the door. He had to wait for a police escort, so that the cops could play the heavies—the worst thing a star can do is to smash through a crowd of admirers. That incident symbolized the entire year: Here was the world's fastest man, and he couldn't move two steps.

After we returned to Toronto, Ben declared that he wanted to go to St. Kitts for rest and recuperation. I wasn't wild about his leaving before his rehab was completed. Dr. Astaphan was away in Europe to work with an Italian sprinter, and Ben wanted no part of Waldemar's intensive treatments while he soaked up the sun. Without the physio's hands-on follow-up through the next few weeks, there could be no guarantee that Ben would recover completely. (While muscle injuries heal rapidly, the trick is to avoid the formation of scar-tissue adhesions. Since these adhesions are both stronger and less supple than the surrounding tissue, they make the athlete prone to new muscle tears adjacent to the original injury site.) But Ben was adamant, and after Desai agreed to keep an eye on him in St. Kitts, I had to let him go.

Ben returned home two weeks later, where he began his season's second six-week steroid cycle and resumed his tempo work to prepare for the early outdoor season. He seemed tentative, his form ragged. While he began to look better after graduating to speed work, I could see he wasn't getting full extension in his injured leg. It didn't help that Waldemar's therapy was interrupted three times by Ben's overseas business trips, two of them to Japan. It took until late April for Ben to begin rounding back to form.

We scheduled his first outdoor race for Friday, May 13th, at an international meet in Tokyo. The opposition was soft; we didn't want Ben to be pressed in his first race, nor could we risk a loss—bad business for the world's top athlete. But Ben had trouble warming up, and by his fifth stride he'd torn his hamstring again, just below the site of the first injury, but worse this time around. Our situation was sliding from serious to dire. After a Japanese doctor confirmed a tear of the hamstring semi-tendiosis muscle, we cancelled the remainder of Ben's early-summer competitions, and aimed instead at our national championships in Ottawa that August. Although the Olympics would be staged later than usual, toward the end of September, our margin of error was fast shrinking.

Back in Toronto, my star and I were again at odds. I wanted Ben to go with us to Europe, where Waldemar could work with him daily. (Astaphan had also agreed to come with us if his expenses were paid.) I was also anxious to initiate some special hamstring rehabilitation exercises, devised by Gerard, which had proven effective in the past. We could begin Ben's treatment on the beach at our first stop in Málaga, Spain, and then use state-of-the-art laser equipment in Formia, Italy.

But Ben dug in his heels. Depressed by the two injuries and frayed by the press of publicity and business, he dreaded the European media hounds and the prospect of being carted from meet to meet. (Ben was especially sensitive about the press at the time, as *The Toronto Star* had just attacked him for his spending habits in an article riddled with inaccuracies.) At a meeting at Ross Earl's house, he grudgingly gave in; he would reunite with the group in Málaga, where our tour would originate. At midnight on the appointed day, Waldemar returned from the Málaga airport with the unsettling news that Ben had missed his flight. Four days later, I received a telex from Dr. Astaphan saying that Ben had just arrived in St. Kitts and would not be coming to Europe after all. While Astaphan's diagnosis and treatment plan (including water-resistance exercises) were in line with those of Waldemar and the Japanese doctor, I was still worried. Astaphan would have no physiotherapist to assist him—certainly no one to compare with Waldemar, who was the best in the business—and I would be unable to supervise the rehab exercises.

Soon after that, my communication with Ben broke down entirely. Our much-publicized rift stemmed from a meeting on June 13th in Padua, Italy, a tour stop where Ben honoured an appearance date. The good news was that Astaphan's treatment had succeeded brilliantly. While Ben's hamstring was not yet fully flexible, Waldemar found no adhesions. Ben's strength hadn't suffered, either, as I saw when he did *ten* bench-press repetitions at 352 pounds. He looked perfectly fit; he'd been working out seven or eight hours a day.

Nonetheless, I was determined to find out where the two of us stood, and finally cornered Ben in his hotel room. It was an awkward meeting, as neither of us was willing to scale the wall that had risen between us. I told Ben that I was upset that he'd failed to stay with the group, as planned. I also chided him for breaching his Diadora contract by dressing in street clothes—rather than his track suit—during an appearance that day. It seemed insane for Ben to put his biggest endorsement at risk.

Ben was visibly agitated—angry with me for not phoning to check his progress in St. Kitts, resentful of Waldemar for failing to anticipate his second injury in Tokyo. Voicing our complaints didn't seem to help. "I don't know how we can work together if you won't listen to me," I said.

"Then I guess we can't," Ben said.

The next day Ben returned to St. Kitts with Astaphan, and I went on to Formia. And that was it—after 11 years, I was no longer Ben's coach. I felt betrayed. How could Ben desert me after all we'd been through together? I felt even worse when the Canadian press portrayed me as a greedy person who cared little about Ben's best interests.

It took me a week or two to sort things out and to realize that many of Ben's grievances were legitimate—even if they had, at bottom, less to do with me than with the impossible pressures that attended the world's fastest human. I'm sure we would have reconciled in any case, but Carl Lewis clinched the deal in Paris later that month. After winning the 100 metres there in 9.99, Lewis put on a protracted show of mugging and bowing. "All I know," Carl announced to the press, "is that I'm running better than ever, and [Ben] isn't running at all."

The showbiz I'd once deemed harmless now vexed me. *There's no way I can let this guy win the Olympics by default—not when Ben is so much better.*

Later that month Ben and I met again at Ross Earl's home in Toronto. We denied the mutual recriminations reported in the press, and picked up where we'd left off. Whatever our differences, I was the only coach he'd ever had, and he was the greatest athlete I'd ever coached. We had a job to do—together.

On to Seoul

Ben returned to action by winning the nationals on August 6th, in a wind-aided 9.90, for the fifth straight year. In a year of unwelcome surprises, I received another one at that time in the personage of Jack Scott, a sport trainer who'd made a career of attaching himself to celebrities, from basketball star Bill Walton to wayward heiress Patty Hearst. After introducing himself, Scott informed me that he had treated Ben's hamstring in St. Kitts with a nerve stimulation machine he was promoting—total news to me. (Dr. Astaphan later confirmed that Scott had treated Ben, but said he doubted it had done much good.)

Two days later, as we boarded a plane in Toronto for Sestriere, Italy, where Ben would run a 9.98 at 7,800 feet, Scott appended himself to our group without invitation. He was nothing if not flexible; the year before, he had claimed to be treating Carl Lewis. When he was unable to get a room near us, he wound up at another hotel—in a room reserved for Lewis, who hadn't yet arrived. (Scott would surface again at the Olympics in Seoul, where he would hover around Waldemar on the days before the 100-metre final.)

On August 17th, Ben met Lewis for the first time that season in Zurich—and finished third in 10-flat to Carl's winning 9.93 and

Calvin Smith's 9.97. It was the first time Carl had beaten Ben in three years, and the American seized upon his victory as a sign of things to come. "The gold medal for the 100-metre race is mine," Lewis proclaimed. "I will never again lose to Johnson."

But I wasn't unduly disturbed by the loss. In fact, I began to feel better about Ben's chances in Seoul—not absolutely certain, as we had been in Rome, but confident. In Zurich I'd seen Lewis, apparently in peak form, run back to his time in Rome the year before, despite the advantage of Zurich's higher altitude and Carl's quicker reaction to the gun. There was no evidence that he had improved. Ben, meanwhile, had been carrying seven extra pounds from his intensive weight work, which had replaced the full-speed sprinting he'd missed since reinjuring his leg in May. After a good start he'd begun to wobble at 60 metres, and Lewis had caught him 20 metres later. Ben's hamstring was healed, but his lack of race preparation had left his quadriceps stiff and unresponsive. He'd looked ragged and tight, weaved about in his lane, and eased up when he saw he was beaten. There was no spring in his stride. In short, Ben had run miserably—and still finished with a time only three or four other men in the world could equal. "If he can run a 10-flat looking that bad," said Manfred Germar, the meet director in Cologne (where Ben again finished third in a cold drizzle four days later), "he'll break the world's record in Korea."

We had five weeks to prove the man right. *Could* Ben run faster than in Rome, where he'd set a mark that some thought would last for decades? Before the recent chaos, we had never doubted it. In a *Sports Illustrated* profile back in November 1987, Ben had projected a 9.78 for Seoul; four months later, he publicly amended his prediction to a 9.79, with all the audacity of Babe Ruth calling his shot by pointing toward the bleachers.

But the strain of that spring and summer recalled another question I had confronted months before: Should we even *try* to go faster? After Rome, a Soviet coach told me he wouldn't push for a personal best in 1988 if Ben were his athlete—there certainly would be less risk of injury for Ben if we held his speed to known levels. The coach had a point, but I couldn't buy it. If we took Lewis's

best reaction time and improved acceleration and added his demonstrated maximum speed, Carl was already capable of a 9.87. Allow
for some moderate improvement, and the margins were too small.
What if Carl were to have a good start and Ben an unusually poor
one? We couldn't sit back and assume that 9.83 would be good
enough forever. The world marches ahead, with you or without you.

At the end, of course, the issue would be settled by those final
weeks of training. Ben would run as fast as he was prepared to
run, no more and no less. After returning to Toronto on August
22 Ben took four days of complete rest and embarked on his final
two-week drug program before the Olympics—three injections
of Estragol and three more of growth hormone. Our scheduling
would provide a 13-day clearance time before a tune-up meet
in Tokyo, which we thought unlikely to be tested, and 26 days
before Ben's final in Seoul—an ample allowance, given our past
experience. (Most other coaches exploited the same window of
opportunity to give their stars one last steroid cycle before the
Games. After the August meets in Brussels and Cologne, the ranks
of top competitors in Europe thinned dramatically, to avoid testing
prior to the Olympics.)

The first positive signs came in the distance drills I'd assigned
to rebuild Ben's speed endurance. The results were electric: Ben
was covering 200 metres in 20-flat, faster than he'd ever run at
that distance, and I knew then he would go no worse than the
low 9.90s in Seoul. The next advance came in Tokyo in early
September, where Ben was drilling at 80 metres—and it wasn't
hard to extrapolate his destination. "By my watch, he's ready to
break 9.90," an Italian reporter exclaimed. I agreed; after watching
Ben's stride, I could tell his quadriceps were far more supple than
in Zurich. With his mechanics back to his normal high level, I knew
Ben was primed for the high 9.80s. "Good," said the Italian, no fan
of Lewis. "I'm going to go tell the Americans he's still injured."

After arriving in Seoul on September 16th, we kept our training
light, as we always did before a major meet; we alternated low
volumes of speed work with days of slower tempo running and
calisthenics. I had never seen Ben quite so fresh. On September

19th, four days before the first two rounds of the 100 metres, he ran close to top speed for the only time that week. He equalled his personal best for 80 metres, and I could see he had more in reserve. Then we proceeded to the weight room, where I supervised Ben in the bench press: four repetitions at 135 pounds, four at 225, four more at 315, and one last rep at 365. Ben's best press ever was 385 pounds, well over double his body weight of 173—unparalleled for a sprinter and competitive with power lifters in his weight class. After he completed the work-out with ease, we discovered we had miscalculated the weights, and that Ben had actually pressed *407* pounds—to the utter amazement of an East German weight coach standing by. "I had heard the stories," he said, "but I never believed them until now."

To deliver a sprinter's personal best, you must bring several components to peak: strength for the start and acceleration, speed for maximum velocity, and endurance to stay the last 30 or 40 metres. Ben's 200-metre runs had proven his staying power. His 80-metre time attested to his speed. And those accidental bench presses showed he was stronger than ever. I was now certain that Ben could run into the low 9.80s, that he would win the gold medal and erase any doubts that he was the fastest sprinter of all time.

As it turned out, I had underestimated him.

I'm not suggesting that our week before the race was a model of cool planning. We were doing just fine on the track, but everything outside spun out of our control. The Olympics are two weeks of excess. There is too much money on the line, and too much fevered flag waving, as though a nation's worth hinged on some 15-year-old's backstroke. There are too many athletes along for the ride. (Few of Canada's 386 competitors had a prayer, and so all the pressure fell squarely on the country's handful of true medal hopes.) And there are too many microphones and tape recorders, each attached to a reporter digging for the smallest scoop, accurate or not. Much of that week in Seoul was lost in rumour and confusion.

The craziness found us as soon as we arrived from Tokyo, after a flight on which Ben was hounded throughout by autograph seekers.

The security in Japan had been unbelievable. They protected the athletes at every turn—there were hundreds of cops in our hotel alone. No one could get near us without our permission. But in Korea it was a different story. The first media platoon attacked at the ramp from our plane, planted themselves in front of us, and walked slowly backwards while firing questions and flashbulbs, forcing us to move at their pace. We got a brief respite in customs, and then I went to check on our luggage while Ben waited behind a screen in a secure zone. Five Korean newsmen met me at the carousel.

"Carl Lewis is scared—I saw it in his face," one of them said. I proposed that Lewis might be less afraid of Ben than of the reporters. (Carl had arrived the day before and had refused to leave the airport until guaranteed safe escort by a phalanx of police.) I asked the newsman how his associates had breached security at the ramp. At that he rubbed his fingers together—the international sign for payola. It turned out that anyone with $5,000 could find out what flight we were on (supposedly a secret) and get their cameras into any part of the airport. I was furious. This was more than a nuisance—it was a serious threat to our safety. Just a few days earlier, North Korean terrorists had issued a threat to kill unnamed stars at the Olympics, and now it appeared that anyone with the price of a bribe could do just that.

The worst was yet to come. To get from customs out of the aiport, we had to walk a narrow corridor, about 5 metres wide and 60 metres long. On either side of us stood a swelling mob of international media, more than 300 people in all, barely contained by some flimsy theatre ropes and a thin line of cops. We'd already announced that we would hold a press conference after arriving at the Olympic Village, but nothing before then. A media liaison said the press would co-operate but asked us to walk slowly, so that everyone could get their photos. We started grimly down this gauntlet, pushing our luggage carts in front of us...and then the dike burst. The people who'd taken pictures at the head of the corridor were now shoving to the end to take more pictures, while those at the end jostled back to hold their positions. Suddenly the ropes came down and we were engulfed by a paparazzi free-for-all. The police were swept aside. An old woman in front of us was knocked to the ground and trampled; her cart was overturned and her bags sent skittering across the floor. Broken camera lenses flew over our heads. I flashed back to Karlsruhe and struggled to stay close behind Ben, keeping my body between the mob and his legs, trying not to step on his feet.

After making it outside, we found that a television crew had beaten us to the Hyundai provided for Ben's arrival. In fact, the cameraman was propped up on the roof so he could film through the windshield, despite a vigorous police clubbing to get him off. The cops threw Ben head first into the car and it squealed away, with the back door still open and those million-dollar legs dangling outside. I was cut off from Ben in the mêlée, and followed separately with our bags.

(As in 1972, security at the Olympic Village was a running joke. At the Seoul Hilton, where the IOC executives were staying, there were metal detectors at the door and mirrors to check the bottom of every limousine for bombs. But the athletes' lives weren't worth as much. After a baggage mix-up at the airport, the American shooting team unknowingly brought 22,000 rounds of live ammunition past the security checks and into the Village. And several members of the media told me they were never searched, even though they had the run of the place.)

After grabbing a yogurt with Ben at the Village cafeteria, I was slammed in the head by a television camera and scalded with coffee. By the time we held our press conference, you could smell the hostility on both sides of the table. The media people were insulted that Ben had told them off at the airport. They were also indignant that Canada's biggest star had declined to march with his national team in the opening ceremonies. I told them I had personally vetoed Ben's participation; it would have kept him on his feet for nine hours and robbed him of a day of training.

After several minutes of the third degree, I went on the offensive. "It was nothing short of a media riot at the airport," I told them. "You've got unprecedented access in this Village, but you have to be responsible. You can't injure the players at the very meet you're supposed to be covering." After I took them to task, the English-speaking press began to blame the Korean media for the trouble—a convenient story, if only partly true.

The conference ended on a more jovial note. When asked if he disliked Lewis, Ben drew a round of laughs by insisting, "I like everyone." Meanwhile, the experts installed Carl as the favourite to repeat in the 100 metres, even though Ben had beaten him in five of their last six meetings. (Las Vegas bookmakers offered 10-1 odds against Ben.)

As race day approached, the Lewis camp revived its campaign to have Ben's record in Rome thrown out for an alleged false start, even though Ben's reaction time had met the accepted limit of .120 seconds. At a coaching clinic in Seville, I'd heard Carl's coach, Tom Tellez, claim that Ben was beating the starter by lifting his hands from the track before the gun. Ben would then remain airborne until the gun fired, Tellez continued, at which point his feet would begin to exert pressure on the blocks. It was a preposterous theory, a physical impossibility—an affront to both Ben and Isaac Newton. The protest should have been moot, in any case, since the rules state that the starter is the only arbiter as to fair and false starts.

(In *Inside Track*, the Lewis autobiography published in the spring of 1990, Carl reprised this complaint, charging that Ben "lifted up with his arms and body quicker than anybody else, but apparently was able to maintain pressure against the blocks as he did so.... No false start was detected by the electronic device [in Rome], but it still should have been called." Here Carl made a fundamental error: A sprinter's start is defined not by the moment he breaks contact with the blocks, but rather by the point when he exerts enough pressure on the blocks to trip the device.)

To our consternation, the Lewis camp had enough clout to pressure the IAAF into an official review of Rome, an unprecedented act. If the protest prevailed and the record was expunged, the psychological pressure against Ben might be insurmountable. If his best start were to be deemed unacceptable, he would have to hold back in Korea, since two false starts would disqualify him. I was

relieved when the IAAF affirmed Ben's record, just three days before the first heats in Seoul, but the episode still rankled me. Would
Carl's tactics get to the starter at the Olympics? We would know
soon.

I never discussed this commotion with Ben, who was already
neck-deep in rumours. There was the story that he was hobbled by
a heel injury. (He actually had bursitis around his right Achilles
tendon—a painful condition, but controllable with a small dose of
cortisone into the bursa.) Another hot report claimed he had left
Seoul for home before the race. (Ben had moved to the Hilton from
the Olympic Village. A security guard watched him leave in a taxi,
then sold the "story" to a Korean newspaper.) The most shameless
media gossip had Ben's father dying in Hurricane Gilbert, which
was raging in Jamaica. (Ben's father came through the disaster
untouched, although his emergency duties as a telephone lineman
prevented him from flying to Korea for the race.) A less single-
minded athlete might never have survived that week.

After the Rome record controversy was settled, Lewis turned
his attention to the U.S. men's 400-metre relay team. He and his
manager, Joe Douglas, began feuding with relay coach Russ Rogers
over the team's composition, to the point where practices were
disrupted. The situation got so bad that Rogers threatened to kick
Lewis off the team—"He's at the end of his rope; the only thing
he can do is hang himself," Rogers said—while head coach Stan
Huntsman publicly ordered Douglas to stay away from the team's
training sites. The Americans, who had won the gold and set a world
record in the event in 1984, were eventually eliminated by a bad
baton pass in the preliminary heat.

I couldn't follow Ben to the Hilton, since I had eight other
athletes to supervise in the Village. But I approved of Ben's
decision to relocate. He needed to focus on his job, with as few
distractions as possible. And the Olympic Village was no place to
do it.

The Village had its pleasant aspects; at times it resembled a class
reunion. I remember Angella exchanging family pictures with a

Kenyan middle-distance runner named Mary—they'd both had babies. Mary was retiring after the Olympics, and she'd brought a small gift for Angella. After eight years together on the international circuit, they knew that this meeting would likely be their last.

But at other times the Village was a zoo of more than 13,000 competitors and uncounted coaches, trainers, and national officials—not to mention the ever-present media, busy contriving stories with an "international friendship" accent. One afternoon, Ben stopped on the street to greet a pretty Italian long jumper. The next day, the Italian papers had them engaged—prompting a furious phone call to the girl from her fiancé. The athletes, meanwhile, were understandably on edge, and—with practice workloads reduced this close to competition—had energy to burn. At one point I checked in on two of my sprinters and found their room knee-deep in fire-extinguisher foam. The perpetrator was Australian quarter-miler and notorious wild man Darren Clark, who'd already made his mark in Seoul by parading through the Aussie women's dorm in a gorilla mask.

Even here, among the most select athletes in the world, Ben was a celebrity. At the track, Ben couldn't sit down to stretch without being surrounded by autograph seekers; a few athletes even asked for mine. Ben's reputation could also work for him in more practical ways. As we were about to flag a taxi to his room at the Hilton, he proposed a bit of mischief: "Let's see if we can get a free car." We crossed the street to the motor pool, where hundreds of Hyundais sat idle, on reserve for IOC executives. Ben was immediately recognized and fussed over by the car jockeys, and several autographs later we had a chauffeured ride to the hotel.

After Ben moved to the Hilton I saw him only on the track, for two or three hours per day. It was after the fact that I learned he'd been in a bar with two women after midnight Thursday—or about five hours before he had to get up on the day of his first two heats. I wasn't surprised to hear he'd been out carousing. Ben liked beer and he loved women, but his nightlife never seemed to hurt him. His metabolism was so high that I never saw him with a hangover, nor did pre-race sex (his fears before Rome notwithstanding) affect his performance. At one Grand Prix meet, a female manager for a world-ranked sprinter kept Ben in the sack until 45 minutes before the race. When it was over Ben jumped into a taxi, took a brief warm-up, and then blew out the field. After the race, the manager needled her beaten runner: "I did my job, but you didn't do yours."

Sprinters are high-strung by nature, like thoroughbred horses, and have more than their share of nervous energy. It may hurt more than help to bottle them up. At the 1982 Commonwealth Games, Mark McKoy decided he'd try something different. He went to bed early and stared at the ceiling, and he got so hyper that he barely qualified the next morning. The following night he said the hell with that, and played cards with his buddies till 3:00 A.M. The next day he broke his personal best in the 110-metre hurdles, won the gold medal, and set a Commonwealth record.

A few days before Ben's final, a well-known Western European official approached me at the warm-up track and asked if I had anything that might help one of his country's top female athletes. The woman had been set back by injuries before the Olympics, the official explained, and wasn't as ready for the Games as she'd hoped. I set up a meeting at the Hilton with Astaphan, the official, and the athlete. The woman told us she'd been stacking Stromba (oral stanozolol), Primobolan (another steroid), and 50-milligram shots of aqueous testosterone daily for several years, in addition to regular doses of amphetamines on competition days. Then she asked us if we had any Dexedrine or Benzedrine she might take for the Olympics. Astaphan and I were shocked; the doctor had planned on offering her nothing more potent than inosine, a legal and mildly anabolic substance. I asked the woman how she could use amphetamines and still pass her drug test. She replied that she routinely evaded her home country's random-testing program by infusing clean urine into her body with the aid of a makeshift catheter—a West German bubble-making toy—and planned to do the same in the Olympics.

At the same meeting, the official told Astaphan and me about an East German star who apparently relied on a similar technique. A functionary had passed the athlete a bouquet of flowers after she won a medal at one major championship and just before she entered the doping control room. When our official spotted a catheter among the blooms, he said, he called it to the attention of an IAAF representative, who backed away from the scene and out to the in-field, where he couldn't be followed.

At less important competitions, tests were so loosely administered that even bolder stratagems could be used. A few months before the Seoul Olympics, I discovered how one star female sprinter evaded meet testing throughout Europe. Whenever the sprinter had to produce a specimen, her coach told me, she would ask a hotel maid to fill the urine bottle, which would then be spirited into the doping control room. As long as the maid was off steroids, the coach added, there were no problems.

The Heats

On Friday, September 23rd, my alarm watch woke me at 6:00 A.M., Seoul time—less than four hours before the first round of heats for the 100 metres. I'd slept with my window half open, and the morning was excruciatingly cold. I ran for the single shower to beat the other Canadian coaches—seven of us were sharing a spartan, four-bedroom apartment at the Olympic Village, complete with paper sheets—and then piled on two sweat tops and a jacket.

I was in luck. The single elevator was available, for a change, saving me a 12-flight walk to the lobby. The Canadian Olympic Association had followed its typical housing assignments: officials on the ground floor; the favoured swim team just above them; then the gymnasts, boxers, shooters, and the rest; and finally the track team on the top floors. The higher your room, the lower your status—which meant that our runners would drain their batteries trudging up and down the stairs.

I headed for the cafeteria, a bit grimly. The International Olympic Committee subscribed to the same service philosophy as the big supermarket chains: Provide enough staff to avert a riot by frustrated customers, but no more. Up to now I'd dodged the hour-long food lines by grabbing some yogurt or fruit salad, but the lines were much smaller now that the events had started, and I got my bacon and eggs—my first hot meal of the week—within 10 minutes.

On the bus to the stadium, a couple of miles away, it was cold enough for the athletes' breath to fog the windows. I arrived at the warm-up track at 7:30, concerned that Ben might be late, but he was waiting for me; he'd been escorted early from the Hilton by Don Wilson of the Royal Canadian Mounted Police and three or four security guards. Seoul had a first-rate warm-up facility, far better than the one in Los Angeles four years before. The area had its own set of stands, and the check-in tent was only a short walk away from the main stadium. We decided to move Waldemar and his massage table to the far side of the track, the first part to be touched by sunlight. Ben seemed extremely relaxed and confident as he lay on the table. When Desai came in around 8:00 the pair jogged two laps around the grass in-field to get the kinks out.

I checked the final starting lists for the initial heats, the first of four rounds spread over two days. There were 13 of them—an unusually high number, as major games rarely have more than eight, and a testament to the 100 metres' standing as the most universal and competitive event in all of sport. More than 100 runners were entered (from 71 nations), of whom 39 would advance to the quarter-finals that afternoon, 16 to the next day's semi-finals, and eight to the finals. We knew pretty well who would make it through. Although the entries were all champions in their own right, and most could run faster than Jesse Owens in his prime, only five or six had any shot at a medal.

The heats would begin at 9:50 and proceed at five-minute intervals. Ben was running in the eighth heat (a fair break for us, since the cold would abate by then), and Desai in the tenth. Though neither would have to run hard before the semis, we scheduled 80-minute warm-up periods for each, including a light, slapping massage.

A week before, Waldemar had performed a deeper massage to lower Ben's muscle tone—the proportion of fired (or contracted) muscle fibres to unfired fibres. Each warm-up and race increases the tone, and the physiotherapist's job in a multi-round meet is a tricky one: If the tone is too high for the early heats, there won't be enough fibre left to contract for an optimal run in the finals. But if the tone is too low, the athlete won't get enough elastic response from his muscles to make it out of the heats and *into* the finals. Even worse, a runner who pushes too hard with low tone risks injury. Ben was so fast that he had some margin for error; he could run pretty damn quick with low tone if he had to. In any case, Waldemar pronounced his tone perfect, with good "rebound." That made me a happier coach, since I still had some anxiety about Ben's rehabilitated hamstring.

I entered the main stadium four heats into the round, and took a seat in the athletes' section, across from the 30-metre line. It would be hard to see who finished where from that point, much less judge the runners' form, but I wasn't anticipating drama that day. The chill air was warming by the minute, as the sun rose above the edge of the modern stadium: good weather for sprinters, who liked it better the hotter it got. All that was missing were the fans. In contrast to Los Angeles, where the early heats had packed them in, the stands were barely a quarter full. With the turnout so sparse, it was all too easy to hear the rhythmic cheers of some two thousand children stationed near the starting line, led by teachers who clearly knew nothing about track. The kids yelled right through the starting commands—an incredible distraction for the runners, especially the nervous ones who weren't sure they would qualify.

I glanced down at the new Rekortan track, a springier surface than the Mondo track in Rome. You can bull over the relatively firm Mondo, relying on sheer power and chopping your stride for greater frequency. But you can't fight against Rekortan—you have to let the track do its thing. A softer track doesn't bounce back, or "return" to your foot, as quickly. If your stride fails to stay full and long, you will quickly go out of phase with the surface; the least tightening in your form will destroy your rhythm. Five years ago that might have been a problem for Ben (and an advantage for the fluid Lewis), but no longer. Ben had learned to relax with the best of them. Of course, it's a lot easier to relax when you're so far in front that you can't see anyone behind you.

As I watched and waited for Ben's race, my main concern was the Korean starter. In one heat the crowd's noise provoked a false start, but the starter blamed it on an athlete. In another heat, a runner fell in his blocks, and Britain's John Regis—who'd been a good bet to reach the semis—paused beside him, assuming they'd be called back. But the starter let the race go, and Regis was out of luck. I didn't like either decision, but I sympathize with starters. With so much at stake, they operate under killing pressure, like air traffic controllers with no back-up. Two days before the opening of a previous Olympic Games, the head starter suffered a nervous breakdown and had to be replaced.

When the eighth heat entered the starting blocks, Ben assumed his typical wide stance, with his hands spread across the width of his 42-inch lane. His dark frame coiled within his singlet and shorts in red with white trim—Canada's colours. Aside from his musculature, which belied his modest body weight, Ben was set apart by two trademarks: his black and yellow Diadora shoes, and the gold chain he always wore around his neck. The gun fired and he powered away from the outclassed field. At 30 metres he shut down his acceleration. At 60 metres he was so far in front—a good eight metres—that the crowd laughed to see it. He virtually jogged through the last 20 metres, almost stopped at the finish line, and still ran a winning 10.37. I felt simultaneously relieved and—as always—amazed at Ben's reserve.

Desai also won with ease, in 10.24. Lewis took the final heat in 10.14, but seemed stiffer than he had in his first heat in Rome, when he'd logged an effortless 10.05 with a legal tailwind. He was following his usual strategy—to intimidate people with superior times in the early heats. Our approach was different. We wanted Ben to conserve his energy for the finals, and so far we were doing even better than in Rome, where Ben's first-heat time had been 10.24. Rome was my reference point, as it had been all summer. Ben, too, had been visualizing that record race for days now, to imprint it on his muscle memory.

Two hours later, my nervous stomach was rebelling again. When the lists for the six quarter-finals were posted, after a delay that cost us our practice starts, I found that Ben had landed in a stacked race. In each of the other heats, there was no more than one major athlete with a shot at the finals. But the second quarter-final had three—besides Ben, there were Linford Christie and the young American Dennis Mitchell. Ben would have to beat at least one of them to be safe, as only the top two finishers in each quarter were assured of spots in the semis, to be joined by the four other sprinters with the best times overall. Ben's coasting was over at this meet. (The tough draw was created by a computer placement which drew the quarter-finals strictly according to the runners' times in the heats, regardless of how high the athletes might have ranked. Since both Ben and Mitchell had run relatively slowly in their heats, they were thrown in against Christie, who had run well.)

I couldn't help thinking about the 1980 Games in Moscow, when defending Olympic champion Hasely Crawford had been jammed into an unbelievably difficult quarter-final with four first-hand winners, while the Russian sprinters were steered into three easy races. Crawford was eliminated—even though he finished faster than any of the Russians.

Just before Ben checked in for his race, I told him not to take any chances—that he needed to put out enough to finish no worse than second. He started beautifully and looked extremely easy when he passed me at the 30-metre mark. But he slowed at 60 metres—*too soon, damn it*—and Christie and Mitchell were coming on. Had they nipped him at the wire? It was hard to see the finish from my angle, but I heard a single dread word from a French coach behind me: "Beaten." In the replay on the big screen behind the stands, my fears were confirmed: Christie had won in 10.11, Mitchell was second in 10.13, Ben had run third, in 10.17.

People were going berserk. I felt dazed. I was sure Ben had understood my pre-race briefing. Was his leg bothering him? Was there some new problem? And there was one other, most urgent question: Would he make the semis? Since he'd run in the first quarter-final, I had to sweat out the remaining five heats before I'd know for sure.

I felt a bit better after Ben's time stood as the best among the non-automatic qualifiers. Back in the warm-up area, I left him alone as Waldemar gave him a post-race rubdown. Ben wasn't all that communicative under the best of circumstances, and he might conceal anything that would make me worry. The worst thing I could do was to panic him. Besides, the semis and finals were just one day away. If Ben had been hurt, his Olympics were over—with or without my hysterics.

As Waldemar continued his work, Lewis surfaced in the warm-up area. A group of schoolchildren in blue uniforms called Carl's name from the stands, coaxing him over, but Lewis had another idea. He walked the length of the track, toward the grassy patch where Waldemar's table abutted the far end of the stands. The children followed and Lewis signed autographs within three feet of Ben's prone body, looming over him for two minutes or more. For Lewis, who had won his quarter in a smooth 9.99 and was doubtless exhilarated by Ben's apparent problems, it was yet another in a series of mind games. "Wise guy," Ben muttered after the incident. "Let's see what he does tomorrow."

(While annoying, Lewis's antics were mild compared to the psych-outs pulled by past Olympic sprinters. At the Montreal Games in 1976, Hasely Crawford, the powerful and volatile ex-machinist, was eating lunch in the Village dining room when confronted by several American sprinters. They made the grave error of telling Hasely they intended to kick his ass. Crawford jumped up toward the intruders, screaming obscenities and knocking his table and plates to the floor with a crash. "When they stepped back from me, I knew they were done," noted Crawford, who went on to win the gold medal. Of course, Lewis knew better than to get up in Ben's face like that. Ben would plough him in the head if he tried. He'd *kill* the guy—you looked at Ben and you knew it.)

On the bus back to the Village, Waldemar told me Ben's muscles felt fine—a touch tight in the calves, perhaps, but he would loosen them up at the Hilton that night. The tone should be excellent for the next day. But I couldn't stop worrying. Waldemar's massage table had lost a wheel, and as I carried it the mile from the bus stop to the physio's room, I replayed Ben's race every step of the way. It was the lowest point yet of a nerve-racking week.

It was only after the final that Ben told me what had happened in his quarter-final heat. He was running fine, he said, but misjudged and shut down a little early. By the time he realized that Christie and Mitchell were on his shoulder, it was too late—and physically risky—to reaccelerate. Ben had scouted the other heats before the race. He knew he was running below 10.20—he'd always had an eerie ability to gauge his own time—and he knew that no one below the top two in any other heat could go that fast. And so, with the licence of genius, he just ran through. (As it turned out, Ben had been conservative; the next-fastest wild-card qualifier ran a 10.26, and the cut-off for the semis was 10.33.) While those around him lost years off their lives, Ben never blinked. He knew exactly what he was doing.

Saturday, September 24th, would be the day of reckoning for Ben and Carl Lewis, now the consensus favourite. It was another chill blue morning, but the day's heat would settle in before the races, as the semis were scheduled for noon. The top four finishers from each would move on to the final, at 1:30 P.M.

When I reached the warm-up track, Ben and Desai—who'd won his quarter-final in 10.16—had finished their jog and were sprawled on the grass. At 8:45, Waldemar treated Ben's sore heels with some anti-inflammatory creams and electronic muscle stimulation. I asked Ben if the heel was a problem; he replied that he would just ignore any soreness. I knew better than to press the point.

I'd had some concern that Ben's heat might be stacked again, but the semis were evenly drawn. Lewis would run first, with his closest competition coming from Calvin Smith, the former world-record holder. Ben would replay his quarter in the second semi, facing Christie and Mitchell again. He'd have to respect them after yesterday, but there were no easy races at this point, anyway. After a couple of practice starts, Ben moved toward the check-in tent 20 minutes before the heat, and I found a seat in the stands.

Lewis's heat began with a false start, one of many in this competition. It didn't help that the Korean "set" command required two syllables instead of one, which threw many runners off balance—though it wasn't so bad as in Finnish, where "set" translates into *four* syllables, practically a dinner speech. According to Lewis, the International Olympic Committee had promised that the "holds"—those tension-filled moments between the set command and the gun—would be slow in Seoul, on the long side of the accepted 1.8- to 3.2-second range, a policy designed for maximum fairness. The U.S. Olympic trials and several European meets had used slow holds to prepare the runners for the Games. But the Korean starter, Lewis charged, was inconsistent—sometimes firing the gun quickly after the set command, sometimes slowly. I agreed with Carl, but my first concern was that the starter simply use common sense in calling false starts. I'd seen precious little of it up to now.

The second start in Lewis's semi was clean, and Carl won going away in 9.97, with a legal tailwind. Though Lewis's form looked good to me, he later told John Smith, the American who had trained with me in 1980, that he hadn't accelerated the way he'd wanted to.

Now Ben was to the line. My nerves had entered the cold-sweat stage. Ben's true state of readiness would soon be revealed. To the world he seemed so fearsome, a sculpted running machine, but I always felt a brief surge of panic before every big race, a small moment when I watched Ben's lane and saw a bony 15-year-old in scruffy black high-tops. How could we go up against these superstars? And then the moment passed, and the boy fleshed out into the imposing man who made all the *others* so nervous, and I remembered how far we'd come....

The starting gun sounded, echoed quickly by the recall gun. Brazil's Robson da Silva had false-started, and the eight sprinters regrouped. The second start was a beauty. Ben went to the front at once, far clear of the others, when—unbelievably—the recall gun sounded again. An official walked over to Ben's lane, and turned on the red light bulb behind his blocks, indicating a false start. The fans booed loudly—*they* knew the start had been fair. Ben couldn't contain his anger. Hands on hips, he glared daggers at the white-jacketed starter, then waved scornfully and paced 15 metres behind his blocks to gather himself. This upset me even more, since Ben couldn't afford to lose his concentration, as he had after his false start in Zurich. Now he'd be running with an acute handicap. It was bad enough to be called back for a real false start. It was much worse to be tagged for a fair start, which tells the sprinter he won't be permitted to get away to the best of his ability.

Once again, the eight runners were set. Once again, the gun sounded—and Ben proceeded to run the most spectacular race of his life. He visibly paused in his blocks, giving everyone else a head start. They went, then he went, as if he were telling the starter: There's no way you'll get a chance to screw me again. After 20 metres he was close to a metre behind the pack. *Time to move*, I thought. *You aren't chasing a bunch of schoolboys here.* And then Ben moved—no, he erupted. He *smashed* the field in the middle of the race. By 40 metres he'd caught up, by 80 he was two metres in front, and from there he coasted across the finish line. I checked the clock: 10.03 into a 1.2-metre headwind. The wind was worth at least a tenth of a second. Ben's late start cost him another tenth, and his easing at the end lost half a tenth. In other words, Ben had run the equivalent of a 9.78—science-fiction time.

To those in the know, Carl Lewis was no longer the favourite for the 100-metre finals. Despite their deceiving semi-final times, Ben had clearly run better—and Lewis, who had watched Ben's race on a monitor under the stands, now knew what he was up against. The fastest man was headed squarely toward a new world record.

As soon as the heat was over, IOC officials clambered down to the in-field, demanding an explanation from the starter. What the hell was going on here? A few minutes later I got the official word: Ben had set off the electronic sensors in the starting blocks (and the alarm in the starter's earphone) by twitching before the gun. The starter had certainly blundered, since twitches are common and should have no bearing on a race. There had been two reasonable alternatives to a recall. Since all the athletes had been motionless after the alarm, the starter could have asked them to stand without charging anyone for a false start, then returned them to the blocks. Or, even better, he could have ignored the alarm, relied on his eyes, and declared a fair start when the gun went off half a second later. As long as everyone moved together, he should have let them go.

While the post-mortem was not exactly reassuring, I was half-satisfied. The starter had surely been put on notice, and like a baseball umpire who makes a bad call, he'd be careful not to repeat his mistake. Back at the warm-up track, Ben said he'd felt good in the semi but was worried about the starter. I told him to forget about it—the last thing I wanted was for Ben to hold back in the finals.

As in Rome, Ben was poised to match Lewis's top speed in Seoul—to go as fast as 40 feet per second. But even though he had grown far beyond the one-dimensional runner portrayed by the press, Ben's entire race was still set up by the tremendous forces he generated at the start. As he liked to say, "When the gun go off, the race be over." It wasn't just that he gained a quick edge at the gun, though he usually did. Ben's advantage was that his superior early acceleration—those first three propulsive strides— allowed him to enter each 10-metre split at a higher velocity than his competitors, until he stopped accelerating at about 60 metres. The gain was exponential, expanding with each stride, as the world would see most graphically in the big race to come.

Desai Williams had also made the final by finishing fourth, in 10.24, in the Lewis semi. Desai was rightfully thrilled. For him the Olympics were already a success, and anything more was gravy. For Ben and myself, however, the ultimate test—of his talent, my methods, and our 11 years of work together—remained ahead of us.

The Opposition

One and a half hours to kill before the big event. Ninety minutes before the most intense—and bitter—rivalry in track would climax in front of the largest audience ever to watch a race: more than a billion people across the planet. The stakes were high for the media as well as for the runners. A Japanese television network paid tens of millions of dollars for exclusive national coverage of the 100 metres alone—as much as a rival network, which sold the rights, had spent for the entire Olympics. A French camera crew set up by the finish line at 2:00 A.M. and proceeded to wait more than 11 hours for 10 seconds of action. This was *the* super-confrontation at Seoul, the race that would make or break the Games.

Unable to find a seat in the athletes' section, I had to cajole my way past a guard to squeeze precariously onto a landing in the press section, nearer the finish line. (Seating is a perennial problem for track coaches at international meets. While other sports—swimming or gymnastics, for example—honour coach and athlete credentials only for their own people, the athletes' section for track and field events is thrown open to the other sports as well. Since track coaches are typically delayed by last-minute warm-ups, they are shunted to inferior seats, if they get seats at all. They often opt to watch their athletes on monitors in the warm-up area instead.)

Though the talk was all of Ben and Carl, aficionados realized that this field was the toughest ever assembled for the 100 metres—an assessment borne out when four of the eight runners finished under 10 seconds, which had never happened before. I'd checked the list and was happy to find Ben in Lane 6, toward the centre of the track. Like most runners, he preferred to be in the middle of things, rather than on the far outside. As I mulled the roster, lane by lane, I saw there wasn't a weak man in the race. The finalists were all shapes and sizes, and while Ben's five-foot-ten physique worked well for him (tall enough for good top speed, compact enough for an explosive start), the field demonstrated that there was no one ideal body type for a sprinter. It reminded me of Abraham Lincoln's response when asked the optimal length of leg for a man: "One that reaches from the crotch to the ground."

Lane One: Robson da Silva, Brazil, a personal best of 10.00. The wiry da Silva was better at 200 metres, at which he'd win the bronze at Seoul. He was a good finisher but a poor starter, and his best 100 time, run at altitude in Mexico City, was equivalent to a 10.11 at sea level. Brazil had a fair tradition in sprinting, but provided little support for its athletes, either financial or technical. I'd worked with da Silva on the Americas' relay team at the World Cup several years ago, and found him cheerful and co-operative, though his English was little better than my Portuguese.

Lane Two: Raymond Stewart, Jamaica, 10.08. Another lanky six-footer, Stewart was Jamaican-born but now attending Texas Christian University in Texas. He was a likeable fellow, easy-going for a sprinter, whose lilting accent was even heavier than Ben's. He and Ben had grown close and often warmed up together, or played dominoes at night. A former NCAA champion and an outstanding finisher, Stewart had run his fastest 10-metre section in Rome (where his personal best had given him the bronze) over the last 10 metres of the race—an unusual feat of speed endurance. Had he been healthy, he would have been a serious medal threat. Unfortunately, a strained quadriceps had hurt his times this year. Since Jamaica had no physiotherapist at Seoul—another example of how Third World athletes are disadvantaged at the Olympics—Stewart got help from Waldemar before the semis.

Lane Three: Carl Lewis, United States, 9.93. A novelist could not have drawn two more different characters than Ben and Carl, born just six months apart. Ben came out of rural semi-poverty in Jamaica, where he raced his friends barefoot in the streets; Carl grew up in an upper-middle-class household in New Jersey and took cello lessons. Ben was a private, direct, sometimes gruff man of few words; Carl could be both garrulous and evasive.

I'd always had tremendous respect for Lewis—on the track. I still consider him the greatest all-round athlete in history, the best 200-metre man, and by far the greatest long jumper. No one has ever performed in three different events at Lewis's level. Only Jesse Owens achieved such overall dominance, but Owens never faced the competition—in either quantity or quality—that Lewis did.

What made Carl great? First of all, he owned a durable, rangy frame, with long and muscular legs. He had terrific technique from the beginning—not surprisingly since both of his parents were track coaches. (He got his start in track at age seven—in contrast to Ben, who'd never worn a pair of spikes until he was 15.) Lewis also had an innate sense of how he needed to train, and of what was good for him, even if that clashed with the notions of his coaches. His self-absorption served him well as an athlete, by helping him stick to what he knew was in his own best interest. Not least, Lewis had a rare, unwavering faith in his ability. He saw no reason to be tense—he always believed he was the best, even after Ben surpassed him—and so he could always relax, no matter what the situation. In 1982, when Lewis ran the 100 metres at the U.S. nationals, I watched him raise his hands in victory well before the finish—*and before he had passed the two front-runners*. He sensed the rate at which he was closing, *knew* he would get by them. It was rare to see such confidence in action, even among the elite. I would never forget that race.

Lane Four: Linford Christie, Great Britain, 10.03. A monster talent who'd bloomed late and was still getting better. At 6-3, Christie was even taller than Lewis and more muscular as well, in the mould of Ralph Metcalfe, the great American sprinter of the 1930s. Yet another Jamaican-born athlete, he was a big finisher and an improving starter, who'd won the 1986 European Championships in Stuttgart. Christie shared Ben's aggressiveness but was more outgoing, with a commanding sense of humour. He was a mercurial sort who'd had his share of run-ins with the British coaching staff, among others. At the Commonwealth Games in 1986, where he'd finished second to Ben, Christie took offence at a comment I'd made to reporters that one of the 100-metre finalists had false-started, but that it hadn't been called. Christie assumed (mistakenly) that I'd been referring to him, and when our paths crossed at the Village cafeteria he came up verbally swinging. "You bloody wanker!" he bellowed, invoking the supreme British street insult. When the Canadian *chef de mission* mildly observed that he too had seen a false start in the race, Christie was unimpressed: "You're an even *bigger* bloody wanker!" Listening to all of this with interest was an elderly woman at a nearby table. "My, my," she said. "This is so much more exciting than lawn bowling." I thought Christie was definitely ready to go under 10 seconds: a major medal contender.

Lane Five: Calvin Smith, United States, 9.93. Quiet, polite, religious, Smith never had a bad word to say about anybody—which made him stand out in the blustery world of sprinters. He was the least imposing of the finalists, at only 140 pounds, but he'd proven he could run with the big boys. He was one of only four men in the world—along with Ben, Lewis, and Christie—who consistently held form to the tape. On a given day, Smith could beat just about anyone, as he had when he set his world record in 1983. He always delivered his maximum effort, but his erratic training— he'd bounced around from coach to coach—made that maximum inconsistent. Smith had never acquired the money or recognition his performance had merited—in part because his mild personality paled before Lewis's, in part because Lewis was just plain better. Calvin had one idiosyncrasy: When he reached top speed, his head would start to roll from side to side, eventually lolling back like a Hare Krishna's. It was actually a good sign for him, a sign that he was loose.

Lane Six: Ben Johnson, Canada, 9.83. The greatest 100-metre man of all time and, at the age of 26, the fastest man in the history of the world. Aside from his extraordinary physical strength, Ben was tougher mentally than any person I'd ever met, with the gift of absolute concentration. Ben's reserve helped him sustain the tunnel vision required of all great sprinters. The public's doubts, the numbing publicity, Lewis's galling stratagems—none of them ever bothered Ben on the track. And throughout the years he'd remained impervious to the most insidious attacks of all—not the taunts and boasts of your enemies, which can egg you on to do better, but the well-meaning reservations of your friends, who try to protect you by deflating your dreams.

After Ben set his world record in Rome, a psychologist at York University tested him to explore how he handled pressure so well. At one point Ben was asked to check the box beside the most appropriate self-description: "Mild-mannered," "Somewhat Aggressive," or "Aggressive." Ben drew a fourth box on the margin of the paper, scrawled "Very Aggressive" beside it, and checked it off.

Lane Seven: Desai Williams, Canada, 10.16. Immensely talented and a dynamite starter, Desai was the second-fastest man, after Ben, in the indoor 60 metres. But even though he'd improved his top speed to a world-class level since rejoining our team the year before, Desai hadn't progressed as far as I thought he might. He'd been ready to run under 10 seconds for some time, but had never quite put it together. He ran much as Ben had before 1984; after a great start, he'd tighten up at 60 or 70 metres as the Lewis and

Christie types began to gain on him. He'd give in to a natural but deadly impulse: He'd fight like hell and try to do *more*, rather than contain himself and trust his form to carry him through. The fact is that when you reach top speed, you *can't* do more. You can only tighten up—and tight muscles consume up to 100 times as much energy as relaxed ones. Those muscles start working against each other, and deceleration is rapid and irrevocable. I felt Desai could run under 10.05 at Seoul, and wished him the best. At the age of 29, he wouldn't have many more opportunities.

Lane Eight: Dennis Mitchell, United States, 10.03. The youngest finalist at 22 (and the shortest man in the field at 5-8), Mitchell was a solidly built and cocky young man who'd made a dramatic improvement in 1988, and his future looked promising. He'd finished second to Lewis at the U.S. Olympic trials with a wind-aided 9.86. He'd also traded recent wins with Desai, and I thought they might hook up in a race within the race in the two outside lanes.

While the media billed the final as a two-man contest, I saw it more in four tiers: Desai, da Silva, Mitchell, and Stewart, who might well approach 10 seconds but would not run below it; Christie and Smith, who could break the still-magic number, and would fight it out for the bronze; Lewis, who had shown the ability to get under 9.90; and Ben, who stood at his private frontier.

The Start

"When the gun go off, the race be over...."

I've had a lot of nervous times in my life, but nothing can match the last few moments before an Olympic 100-metre final. So much is at stake in so short a time: an athlete's reputation, his commercial future, and his place in history; the vindication—or repudiation—of a coach's theory and practice. From gun to tape, a ten-second race is a study in compression; it is *there* and then it is gone. For most Olympic finalists, the great adventure of their athletic lives goes with it.

In truth, the competition may be even briefer than 10 seconds. A coach can often read the outcome long before the finish line. Some races are decided within the first few steps, or even in the reaction to the gun. In Rome, Ben beat Lewis out of the blocks by sixty-seven thousandths of a second (.129 to .196), and ultimately won the race by one-tenth of a second. He racked up *two-thirds* of his total winning margin before completing a single step.

(As well as he reacted in Rome, Ben could be quicker still. At Cologne in 1984, he logged a reaction time of *.0997 seconds*—the best ever recorded. He had broken through the tenth-of-a-second barrier, a feat long believed beyond human limits. In the process, he set off the starter's pre-set alarm and was called for a false start, even though he hadn't jumped the gun.)

Ben's reaction-time advantage came from both the sheer explosiveness of his nervous reflexes and his unparalleled physical power. A less powerful runner might respond to the gun as quickly, but Ben tripped the sensors faster because his feet pushed harder (at a given point of reaction) against the blocks' sensitive rubber pads, and so he reached the critical pressure threshold that much sooner. Ben's immediate pressure and ultimate pressure were both greater than anyone else's. As a result, he would be first out of the blocks nine times out of ten. His reaction was so violent that he'd often rip his blocks—despite their 16 embedded metal spikes—clear out of the track surface.

In addition to his physical superiority, Ben saved several milliseconds with superior concentration tactics. He inhaled the instant he heard the set command through the speaker in his starting blocks. (Although their sound quality is tinny at best, the speakers are useful in negating the advantage of runners in the inside lanes, who would otherwise hear the starter's commands slightly sooner—given the speed of sound—than those on the outside.) Ben would hold his breath until the next sound triggered him, and then exhale as he pushed off. A runner who continues to breathe between the set command and the gun may get caught in mid-breath—forcing him to stop the breath and *then* exhale and push, an added distraction which delays response.

Technically defined, a sprinter's start consists of his reaction time plus his first three strides. Ben was a natural in this aspect of the game. He had never worked out of the blocks before we got together in 1977, but he took to them right away, and by 1981 he was the best starter in the world. Where the typical sprinter concentrates on driving his back leg forward as quickly as possible, Ben's approach was different. To exploit his great strength and *blast* out at the start, he fixed his back leg in the blocks as he drove out through his huge lower back muscles. (Ben's erectors, the muscles that flank the lower spine, were developed to the size of an average man's forearms, and sometimes lent him the illusion of a hunchback. In fact, Ben had a classic sprinter's swayback.) That rear leg not only pushed sooner and harder than those of his competitors; it pushed *longer*.

As Ben pushed, his torso uncoiled—the primary source of his superior power. Other runners hunched over at the hips during those first strides, in a spinal curve which drained significant force from their forward propulsion. They pulled away and bent their rear knee before the leg had delivered its full force for them. By contrast, Ben achieved a virtual straight line—the most efficient path for power— from his shoulders to his rear foot. He dropped his hips, pushed and extended through his back, and drove out with *both* feet. By the time his rear foot lost contact with the blocks, his front foot was about to come off as well. The result was a zipping, syncopated two-step, each stride measuring a mere 18 inches, the feet landing with the briefest of beats: Ben's leap. His rhythm was so quick that, in most races, he was into his third step while his rivals were still taking their second.

Only a man with Ben's tremendous back strength could force his centre of gravity so far forward. (At his first stride, the angle of Ben's extended body to the ground was 42 degrees.) It pushed even Ben to his limit, to the edge of control and occasionally beyond. In Rome he had stumbled and lurched slightly to his left and then heavily to his right, nearly falling into Lewis's lane. (If he'd actually touched the lanes' dividing line, he could have been disqualified.)

Ben started this way naturally, without any tutoring on my part. The leap startled me the first time I saw it, during a work-out at a Toronto high school in the summer of 1977. Like everyone else, I saw that Ben was doing something different out of the blocks. But I couldn't figure out exactly what it was until I watched him on videotape.

My other young runners started conventionally, and a few of them—notably Mark and Desai—became as good as anyone else in the world. But when I saw that Ben's unorthodox technique worked for him, I decided not to monkey with it—despite the unsolicited advice of other coaches. "Ben starts funny," they'd tell me. "Why don't you fix it?" Then, after Ben started winning big, they turned around and began asking their sprinters to copy him. They were wrong both times. Nobody should copy anybody; everyone should do what they do best. Less powerful runners couldn't use such an extreme set position to good effect. Ben's advantage was untranslatable.

All coaches have their own theories about technique. The best know when to adapt their theories to the idiosyncrasies of their athletes. In short, they know when to shut up.

It would be soon now. The tailwind was rated at 2.5 miles per hour—about half the legal limit, the same as in Rome—and the temperature was a balmy 25 degrees Centigrade (or 77 degrees Fahrenheit): near-optimal conditions. My shirt was damp, nonetheless, with the sweat of anxiety. The eight finalists, now warm and limber, were asked to take their places: "On your marks!"

Elsewhere in the stadium, a Soviet and a Bulgarian duelled for the gold in the triple jump. At two pits at the south end, high jumpers alternately stretched and loped toward the bar in hopes of qualifying for the next day's finals. But all eyes were now locked on the straightaway along the east side of the clay-coloured track, where the eight fastest men in the world would be unleashed.

There was gamesmanship to the last. As his opponents settled themselves into their starting blocks, Ben lay a few yards back. In past races, Lewis had deliberately delayed his move to the blocks, as a ploy to keep other runners waiting and perhaps to fray their nerves. This time Lewis stalled once again, but Ben waited even longer, and was last of all to enter the blocks, with his right foot set a foot-length behind his left and about a metre behind the starting line. He lined his heels flush with the block pedals, where they would stay until the gun: one less variable to worry about. He spread his arms to the far edges of his lane, with fingers splayed at the white-painted lines. Ben's stance was wider than any other world-class runner. It allowed him to lower his upper torso and his centre of gravity, and in turn furnished more thrust when he uncoiled—a distinct advantage for an athlete strong enough to exploit it.

"Quiet at the start, please," asked the public address announcer, and the crowd hushed to an unnatural stillness: the lull before a bomb drops. Lewis settled into his blocks in lane three. I stood on my toes, peering between reporters' heads for the best possible view.

"Set!" Ben inhaled and smoothly raised his hips, the only adjustment he needed to make. His wide hand spacing helped him find a comfortable and motionless set position, with his weight far enough back to keep his heels on the pedals. Less prepared sprinters might still be fidgeting in their blocks—or, if their hips rose too sharply at the set, they might pull their feet off the pedals. If caught by a fast gun, they were then forced to rock their weight back to the pedals before they moved forward—a fatal waste of time and power. Not only would they be moving backward while their opponents were moving forward, but they would also have to fight the inertia of their body's reverse motion—a far greater impediment than inertia at rest. They might as well be starting with lead weights on their backs.

All eight finalists at Seoul were right-footed—that is, they strode first with the right foot out of the rear block. Even so, Ben stood out in the line. All of his body's angles were more acute: his butt higher above his shoulders, his stomach almost touching his drawn-up left thigh. His head was also fixed higher—a throwback to the Jesse Owens era—to help keep his back straight after the start, against the conventional wisdom that a runner's head should align with his spine. Ben's stance was uniform each time out, a prime factor in the consistency of his starts, no matter how long the hold before the gun.

In those final moments of anticipation (the hold actually lasted about three seconds, considerably longer than in Rome), while I held my own breath in empathy, Ben's eyes gave a single, involuntary twitch as he stared blankly at the finish line. He'd been trained not to dwell on the impending sound of the gun. He concentrated, instead, on what he'd do *after* the gun sounded. Ben ignored his legs and focused only on his left hand, which would trigger his leap. Percy Duncan had taught me this trick back in

1970, to my great benefit, and I in turn had drilled it into Ben until it became second nature. It spelled the difference between reaction and reflex, and could be worth several hundredths of a second.

(As a result of such training, a good sprinter may false-start in reaction to any abrupt noise: a cough, a sneeze, a camera click. When Pierfrancesco Pavoni ran next to Ben in the 1983 World Championships in Helsinki, he false-started after Ben's watch alarm—still set on Toronto time—went off accidentally during their quarter-final. Pavoni, a top contender, got off miserably in the second start and was eliminated.)

Back in my own racing days in the early 1970s, Harry Jerome had insisted to me that sprinting was controlled from the arms. I knew he was right—I could *feel* my acceleration coming from my arms as I ran—but the view was heretical. When I included it in a paper on sprint technique, I was widely criticized. There was no question that the arms must piston at the same frequency as the legs' stride—in Ben's case, up to five times per second. But the experts maintained that the sprinter's body operated in synchrony, with legs and arms in simultaneous action. Years later, neurological research confirmed what I had experienced: that arm action must slightly, almost imperceptibly, precede leg action, and that the arms indeed control the stride. Ben's arm strength—enhanced by rigorous weight training—figured heavily in his success.

Like most of his contemporaries, Ben began by driving that left arm forward with its elbow splayed to the side, a practice innovated amidst controversy by Bob Hayes, the 1964 Olympic champion. The experts of that era insisted Hayes would go even faster if he pumped his lead arm straight forward and in close to his body, in a neat plane like everyone else. But Hayes was right and the experts were wrong. They missed the main point: The object of the exercise was to move the lead hand—from its set position on the ground to the optimal, extended position in front of the sprinter's head—as quickly as possible. There can be no quicker path than a straight line—and the lead hand can move straight only if the elbow bends outward. Hayes' more conventional opponents—much like Carl

Lewis a generation later—lost time because their lead hands swept forward in an arc, rather than in a line.

Here Ben again diverged from the pack. Most sprinters raised their left hand to ear level. Ben drove his hand several inches *above* his head, with far more force than any opponent's, until it stuck up like a flag. That one aggressive left-arm motion prefigured Ben's entire race. He'd taken Percy's old concept and made it over in his own explosive image. I had never seen anything like it.

Now I was seeing it again, almost as the white-blazered starter squeezed the trigger. The start was clean, and far more even than in Rome. We found later that Ben's reaction time was .132 seconds— the best in the field, but only marginally faster than Lewis at .136 and Christie at .138. (These statistics, as well as the split times cited later in this chapter, were produced by Charles University's biomechanical study of the race.) In contrast to Rome, Ben would gain only 3 percent of his final margin over Lewis at the gun. It was not so much that Ben reacted more slowly in Seoul (the difference was only three thousandths of a second), but that the competition did much better—further evidence that a longer hold allowed more runners to compete at their best. This race would be decided in the running; there could be no complaints about "fliers" from the Lewis camp.

To eyes unaided by digital read-outs, however, it looked as if Ben seized his edge from the very start. While he reacted at par with several others, his subsequent movements were significantly faster. At Seoul, as usual, his left hand came up before anyone else's. And while the others still had their right arm back, at the maximum extension of their initial drive, Ben's right arm was coming down and forward, as he was already into his leap. (Because of his lanky frame and traditional technique, Lewis's lead arm levered most slowly of all.) Ben's superior force from the blocks threw his centre of gravity farther in front of his feet, which made his first three steps much quicker than anyone else's. His first step was down by .4 seconds, his third by .8 seconds—a sequence so sudden that it rocked Ben toward the left side of his lane. Though he was only inches ahead of the field at this point, he had taken his third power stride well before the rest, a decisive advantage in the early going. He had delivered an extra blow against inertia and could begin to channel his power toward the pursuit of sheer speed, while others still struggled with their own mass.

One second into the race, I could see a clear separation between Ben and the pack, which remained in a virtual line. It was a healthy margin, but I wanted *more*. I hated suspense; I wanted Ben's burst to decide matters early. I wanted this race to be over.

The Running

At *10 metres* Ben was already more than a foot ahead of his nearest pursuers—Desai, da Silva, Stewart, and Lewis, with the rest of the field another foot behind. He seemed to pause slightly and gather himself for a stride or two, as if shifting gears, which was typical for him at this stage. Ben may have lost a few inches at that moment, but the gathering capped an initial burst that had gained him much more. It would be the only part of his race that was less than headlong; from here on, he would accelerate continuously to the 70-metre mark.

Ben was a consistent model of correct "sprint position," the technique that I tried to develop in each of my runners, male and female. To hold that position for a full 100 metres requires both confidence (to avoid tightening up) and strong hamstrings (to keep from buckling at the knee when you strike the ground from a higher centre of gravity).

Ben's form had never been better than in this race: head erect; shoulders relaxed; each hand rising to face-level at its apex; full extension of the driving leg, with hips held high. Ben had emerged from his starting crouch and into his erect running position by his fifth stride. His opponents required seven or eight strides to do the same. Another loss of efficiency for them; another edge for Ben.

While other world-class runners might display comparable technique, no one had ever combined such flawless mechanics with so much brute strength. Ben's power made him fastest, but his form was the vehicle for that power. Only one physical detail escaped the ordered mesh of man and motion: the random jiggling of Ben's gold chain.

Most of the stadium spectators were too distant to observe such details. Even on television (before the slow-motion replays), there was too much to be seen in too little time. But the result of Ben's power and form—and his arrival at full sprint position before anyone else—was the expanding sliver of daylight between himself and the pack.

He was already six hundredths ahead of Lewis.

At *20 metres*, I thought the race was over, barring some freak mishap. There was only one question: How expensive had it been for Ben to invest such a massive effort so early—and would it cost him later on? If Ben could match the others' maximum speed and staying power (and his training had assured me that he could), he would not be caught. He was two feet ahead of Desai in second, with Stewart, Smith, and then Lewis all in lock-step another foot or so behind.

I was not surprised by Ben's ability to reach such high speed so quickly. We had honed his early acceleration for years with our cone drills, where Ben began by running a "smooth" 20 metres with a gentle acceleration, then floored it for the next 20, then eased off again. After hundreds of repetitions, a neurological imprinting had occurred. When Ben reached a certain velocity, he automatically kicked into over-drive. Under race conditions, where the initial acceleration was steeper, he reached his over-drive phase at about 10 metres, while other runners were still in first gear.

The result in Seoul was especially graphic. From 10 to 20 metres, Ben's margin over Lewis stretched from six hundredths to nine hundredths, a back-breaking increment. Ben would best Lewis in every 10-metre segment of this race through 50 metres, but the worst beating occurred during their early acceleration.

After the race, Lewis would claim that he was unaware of Ben's huge lead until he looked toward lane six at the 70-metre mark. But Carl is contradicted by the videotapes. They show that he peeked over at Ben three times—and the first time at 20 metres. The glances didn't appear to hurt Carl's form, but they may have affected his concentration. A sprinter wants to lock his eyes on the finish line, to focus only on himself. That was usually no problem for Lewis, a paradigm of self-absorption. But there was nothing usual about this race. Lewis was running superbly, even by his own formidable standards, yet found himself being ground to a pulp.

At *30 metres*, in the wake of Ben's pre-emptive strike, 70,000 people were now on their feet, craning to see a historic race before it passed them by, perhaps sensing that it already had.

Desai remained in second place, though he'd now slipped six hundredths behind Ben. The rest of the field stayed tightly packed, from Lewis and Smith (his head now sagging backwards) at the front, to Christie and Stewart, and finally to da Silva and Mitchell at the rear—all six of them within three hundredths of one another. The only remarkable development was the widening gap—about three and a half feet now—between Ben and the pack. Lewis had routed the field in the 1984 Olympics in Los Angeles, winning by twenty hundredths, but he compiled most of his margin in the last 30 metres, and half of it in the last 10. You just didn't dispose of an Olympic final this early, as if it were some preliminary heat, but Ben was doing just that. What's more, the best was yet to come. At 30 metres, he later remarked, "I blew it out."

Ben's stride was a thing of beauty in this race. In contrast to his form in Zurich six weeks before, he appeared fluid and supple throughout. His renewed flexibility enabled full extension of his hip, knee, and ankle joints, and—more important—allowed him to tuck his heel up tight to his buttocks in the recovery phase of each stride, when the leg is coiling underneath the body and moving forward. In Seoul, unlike Zurich, the ankle of Ben's recovery leg swung above the knee of the supporting leg (the one on the ground). His tighter ankle tuck shortened the leg's lever and allowed the knee to swing forward more quickly. As a result, Ben could stride faster with the same expenditure of energy—and without exhausting his quadriceps, the muscles which tend to tire most over the last 30 metres. In Zurich Ben appeared heavy, even dragging; in Seoul he looked fluid, his motion apparently effortless.

This was not to say that Ben's stride was technically perfect, nor even symmetrical. As always, his left knee drifted out to the side with each driving step. It was Ben's most obvious physical anomaly, but it never impeded him, and I'd resolved long before to ignore it. The human body adjusts to small idiosyncrasies, and you tamper with them at your peril. There are no style points to be won in sprinting. There is no sense in regimenting form if the result is a slower runner.

Ben's margin over Lewis stood at ten hundredths and counting. "By 30 metres, I knew I had won, just like in Rome," Ben told the press after the race. "I sailed right through." Indeed, Ben's official split time at 30 metres was 3.80 seconds—identical to his split in Rome. But on closer inspection, Ben's dominance was even greater this time around. After subtracting reaction times, Ben's actual *running* time in Rome for 30 metres was 3.68 seconds, to Lewis's 3.73—a margin of five hundredths. At Seoul, Ben improved to 3.67, while Lewis *slowed* to 3.76—a difference of nine hundredths. As bad as the race now looked for Lewis, it might have been far worse. Had he reacted as poorly in Seoul as he had in Rome, he would have been almost twice as far behind.

At *40 metres*, Ben continued to pour it on. From 30 through 60 metres, his stride frequency peaked at an average of 5.02 strides per second—comparable to his peak frequency in Rome, and significantly higher than any of his competitors'. Ben was the only world-class sprinter *capable* of exceeding five strides per second—and, most likely, the only one in history to do so. Out of his half-second of total improvement in the 100 since 1981, more than 80 percent had derived from his boosting that frequency. It was the single greatest key to his supremacy. By the end of this race, Ben would take 46.6 strides—or three more than Lewis.

Ben had not yet reached his top velocity, however, because his stride *length* would continue to increase until it levelled off at around 70 metres. At this stage of his career, Ben consistently kept these two basic variables—stride frequency and length—in perfect balance. He knew that any disproportion would be costly. If you force too great a frequency, your stride will inevitably shorten, negating any gain. Worse, you will overload the brain stem, which must isolate the right muscles for work at the right time and prevent interference by their antagonists. The result: You will tighten up. At the same time, if you over-stride for greater length, you'll land too far in front of your centre of gravity, and lose power and co-ordination.

But for Ben, everything was in place, and it was at this stage that his running began to seem gravity-free. After a sprinter's support leg leaves the track, and as his recovery leg comes forward and down, he is completely airborne for far more time than not. (As Jesse Owens once explained, "I let my feet spend as little time on the ground as possible. From the air, fast down, and from the ground, fast up.")

Because he was strongest, Ben recovered from each stride's impact faster than his rivals, and so he spent less time on the ground than anyone else. By 40 metres, his whole torso was moving up through his hips in a phenomenon known as *lift*. He was pushing with so much force that his body moved in two planes at once, both out and slightly up, until he *rose over* the track between his staccato foot taps. Most sprinters' centre of gravity begins to droop shortly after they leave the ground, but Ben's hips continued to ascend well into each propulsive step.

Four feet behind in second place, Desai was still running well, and he'd preserved an edge of four hundredths over Lewis and Smith. But the tapes would show that his form began to waver here—though minutely at this point, and without any apparent cost. He doubtless saw Ben push into over-drive and tried reflexively to respond—his fatal flaw—rather than simply to keep going. It's terribly difficult to maintain one's tunnel vision in a sprint, in part because of a peculiar optical illusion. A runner's peripheral vision "pulls" objects closer to him than they actually are. In this race, Desai's vantage point was a double whammy. As he watched Ben pull away, just one lane to his left, he thought he saw the rest of the pack gaining on him even before they did so.

From a competitive standpoint, the 10-metre segment from 30 to 40 was Ben's second-strongest of the race, after the one from 0 to 10. He gained another three hundredths on Lewis, to go thirteen hundredths ahead of his top threat—or three hundredths more than Ben's *final* margin over Lewis in Rome.

At *50 metres*, Ben's split times began to place his performance into historical perspective. In 1987, Ben set the world indoor record for 50 metres at 5.55 seconds—a phenomenal seven hundredths faster than anyone else had ever run. In Rome, he finished 50 metres in 5.53. At Seoul, his split time was 5.50. Now almost five feet in front, Ben was running a private race against time, drawing inexorably away from both the field and his own world records.

It used to be widely held that a sprinter's acceleration in the 100 metres was virtually complete at the 30-metre mark. There might be a slight upward drift in velocity after that point, according to this view, but the rest of the race was essentially an exercise in maintenance and then deceleration. The bankruptcy of that theory was made plain at Seoul. If you plotted Ben's pace on a graph, you would find a clear rise between 40 and 60 metres. All of the finalists save Stewart were now at or approaching their maximum speed, yet Ben was still pulling away; here was the ultimate vindication of my emphasis on high-speed training. Ben gained another two hundredths over Lewis from 40 to 50 metres, another game-breaking increment in a short sprint. (A typical 100-metre race is won by a *total* of one or two hundredths.) Moreover, those two hundredths were worth far more distance than a similar time gap at the start, since mid-race velocities are so much higher. In these 10 metres, Ben added nearly a foot to his lead. He turned a breakaway into an irrevocable rout.

With Lewis now fifteen hundredths behind—more than two metres, or six and a half feet, and still running third behind Desai— Ben kept stoking the rivalry for his own purposes. It was an act of imagination, for Lewis had fallen outside Ben's peripheral vision. "I said to myself, 'He's coming,' " Ben related after the race, "and I did my best to hold form."

And hold it he did. Each stride was a perfect duplicate of the one before. Ben had entered that state of primal consciousness, a place of utter freedom yet total control. As Harry Jerome had conveyed to me years before, elite sprinters perform in a time warp, in which a 10-second race seems to last far longer. As if in slow motion, they are aware of every step—a sensation that non-sprinters, who run amidst a clutter of struggling body parts, never experience. Like professional pianists, who simply *know* where the keys are, the great sprinters are going too fast to dwell on technique, aside from an occasional spot-check on one or two key components—in Ben's case, his hand position. Any extraneous focus would inhibit them. It would only get in their way.

As Ben hit his top speed, he was totally relaxed. His shoulders were loose. His hands were open, with fingers extended—another harmless mannerism. (Most runners hold their hands slightly cupped, with the thumb and index finger touching as if holding a pencil.) Ben's eyes were half-lidded; he looked as if he were falling asleep. His jaw muscles were so slack that his cheeks rolled up and down with each stride, undulating with impact.

Ray Stewart, meanwhile, began to slow at around 45 metres. By 50 metres he was visibly limping; by 60 he'd fallen hopelessly behind the pack. He had pulled his quadriceps again, and his race was finished. (Despite this mishap, Stewart's star would continue to rise; after the 1989 season, *Track & Field News* would list him as the best 100-metre man in the world, over Lewis, Mitchell, and Christie.)

At *60 metres*, Ben had just completed his fastest 10-metre split. He ran the segment from 50 to 60 at 12.1 metres per second, or close to 30 miles per hour. (Within any given segment, a runner's velocity fluctuates within a narrow range. A runner is always either accelerating or decelerating; according to physical law, there can be no middle ground.) Ben's feet were a blur. In the recovery phase—when a runner's foot moves forward—the heel is travelling almost *twice* as fast as the body, since it is moving from a point behind the torso to a point in front of it. At top speed, Ben's heel moved from zero to 80 kilometres—or 50 miles—per hour and back to zero in *one tenth of a second*—an acceleration rate astronomically higher than that of the fastest Lamborghini.

Between 1986 and 1987, Ben had broken the world record in the 60 metres indoors three times, cutting it from 6.54 seconds all the way to 6.41—truly a quantum leap, especially for such a short race. In Rome he ran this split in 6.38; in the Seoul finals he was timed at a surreal 6.33.

By 1988, Desai had become the second-fastest man in the indoor 60 metres, and he had kept that position to this point in the race, though barely over a ground-swallowing Lewis. The two were followed closely by Christie and Smith (his head now rolling from side to side), with Mitchell and da Silva trailing. Ben's gap over Lewis held steady at fifteen hundredths—an impenetrable advantage, even if Ben were to falter down the stretch. The enormity of that lead made it appear to some that no one else was running very well. In fact, three of Ben's opponents were taking dead aim at personal bests.

At this point, Lewis took his third glance at Ben. To his credit, he didn't panic—his stride remained as long and loose as ever, and he matched Ben's maximum speed of 12.1 metres per second. (The next-fastest maximums were attained by Christie, at 11.9 metres per second, and by Smith and Mitchell, at 11.8.) But Lewis couldn't make up any ground, and he couldn't hide the expression on his face. At 20 metres it had registered confusion; at 40 metres, desperation. Now it bore the stamp of tight-lipped resignation. Lewis was losing the big one, and there was nothing he could do about it.

At *70 metres* Ben's stride length peaked at about eight feet, average for a top sprinter, though shorter than Lewis's, Christie's, and even the smaller Smith's. His exceptional frequency had diminished only slightly, and thus he stayed near top speed. His body was now absolutely erect; he no longer maintained the forward trunk lean that had framed his acceleration. This was a matter of physics. The higher the velocity, the lower the rate of acceleration, until it becomes nil at maximum speed and obviates the need for any lean. At that point the upright runner has the advantage, since his hips can move most freely.

Ben sensed he had the gold medal in his pocket, and that all that was left was a new world record. He would have that as well if he could control his deceleration, and what went with it: the stubbing into the ground, the erosion of form, the gradual increase of contact time between foot and track. All sprinters inevitably decelerate, as no runner can maintain a world-class rate of acceleration for a full 100 metres. In Ben's favour was his great elastic strength— his ability to resist and respond to the shock of the ground and to regroup for a second acceleration phase. (Recent studies at Charles University had confirmed that a sprinter might recover and accelerate *again* up to three times within 100 metres—in a cycle corresponding, perhaps, to breathing patterns.)

Ben's lead now peaked at an improbable sixteen hundredths over Lewis, who'd rolled into second. Christie and Smith followed another three hundredths back, just in front of the fading Desai, with Mitchell and da Silva falling further behind.

At *80 metres*, the historic proportions of Ben's race became most graphic. His split time was 8.02 seconds—nine hundredths faster than his 8.11 in Rome, a record performance that many had believed would outlast the century. His lead over Lewis, who was pulling away from the others, remained at sixteen hundredths— about seven feet. This race would finally kill the old canard that Ben "stole" his races from Lewis with quicker starts and early accelerations, but that Lewis finished better and reached a higher maximum speed. This theory had suffered in Rome, where Ben had first matched Lewis's maximum velocity. But in Seoul Ben went further. He excelled in every phase of the race, from start through acceleration to maximum speed. The electronic split times showed that Ben had either beaten or tied Lewis in every 10-metre segment to this point.

Unfortunately, there would be no way to assess the final phase: Ben's speed endurance over the last 20 metres. It could not be measured because Ben, in another Olympic first, had simply decided to stop running hard. The first sign came at the 80-metre mark, when he stopped driving his arms. His hands now rose only to his shoulders, and the reduced effort promptly weakened his stride.

The only competition was for the silver and bronze. Form would out, as usual. Christie lay in third behind Lewis, followed tightly by Smith. Like Lewis, their strides remained sure, their arms loose and out from their bodies. Desai, meanwhile, had dropped far back to fifth, nine hundredths behind Lewis and barely ahead of Mitchell, and I knew he would not win a medal that day. He was tightening again, trying desperately to keep up, and losing more and more ground as a result. Desai's head seemed to shrink into his hunched-up shoulders. His stride shortened, and his arms pressed in too close; his legs now cartwheeled behind the vertical plane of his torso. For all of his experience and talent, he was reacting like a novice. At this level, Desai still felt he was in over his head.

At *85 metres*, Ben stopped pumping his arms entirely, and began to turn his head toward his left. Both Desai and Mitchell dropped back, Desai more dramatically. Da Silva, the long-winded 200-metre man, steadied for his finish.

At *90 metres*, Ben glanced back and to his left, toward Lewis, who reminded us of just how good he was in defeat. The defending Olympic champion opened up a two-foot lead on Christie for second, with Smith another foot back and holding. Mitchell steadied; Desai fell behind him to sixth.

At *94 metres*, Ben began to raise his right arm in anticipatory celebration and lost whatever residual drive he had left from his backswing. His deceleration became drastic—but he was still six feet in front of Lewis.

At *95 metres*, Christie and Smith began to lean toward the finish line, hoping to shave one or two hundredths off their time. (A sprinter's finish is determined by the instant his torso—not his head or foot—crosses the line.) But they misjudged the line, and by throwing their arms back too soon, they forfeited upper-body power over the last two strides. (Ben never leaned, for this very reason; he saw no point in taking the gamble.) Desai made the same mistake, and aggravated it by turning his head to his left.

Lewis continued to edge away from the leaners, and knew he had clinched the silver. While Carl would later claim that he was happy because he "did the best" he could, he in fact finished at less than his best. With no shot at Ben, he dropped his arms during his last two strides, and neither pumped nor leaned. Carl wouldn't admit it, but for him the Olympics were about winning, above all.

At *97 metres*, Mitchell leaned a bit better and later than Christie and Smith, but couldn't get close to either. Da Silva, who'd made up more than two feet on Desai since the 80-metre mark, timed his lean perfectly, and in this case it made the difference—he would nip Desai at the wire.

Ben's right arm now shot straight up, his forefinger jabbing the air. I know that some fans deemed this an electric moment, a spontaneous celebration by an athlete at his career's climax. I saw it as something else: a taunt aimed specifically at Lewis, the man who had mocked Ben and denied his greatness for so long. (The videotapes show that Ben was glaring straight at Lewis, who returned a sour glance of his own.)

Ben's display upset me even more than it had at Zurich in 1986. Once again the world had lost an opportunity to see how fast the human body could go—and I'd missed the chance to see just how much I'd achieved as a coach. It's still painful to me. At the time,

Ben figured he would reset the world record several times more. He was only 26, after all, and still getting better. But an elite sprinter is in absolute top form for only two or three big outdoor meets each year, and who knew when we'd be favoured again with optimal wind and weather? (I believed that Ben had been ready to set a world record for at least a year before Rome, but we'd been repeatedly frustrated by headwinds.)

At *100 metres*, with his arm still in the air, Ben crossed the finish line after 9.79 seconds, the first Olympic 100-metre champion to break the world record since Jim Hines in 1968. (With its fatiguing series of heats and unrelenting pressure, the Olympics may be the least likely place for sprinters to set a world mark.) He was followed by Lewis, at 9.92; Carl had recovered only three hundredths from 80 to 100 metres, despite Ben's deliberate slowdown. Next came Christie at 9.97; Smith, 9.99; Mitchell, 10.04; da Silva, 10.11; and Desai, 10.11. Stewart limped home in 12.26.

Taken as a group, the numbers were truly historic. For the first time ever, four runners broke the 10-second mark in a single race. Four of the eight set personal bests—including Desai, who made us both proud despite his loss of ground down the stretch. (At the end of the year, *Track & Field News* would rank Desai tenth in the 100 metres; he became my fourth athlete to crack the world's top ten.)

For Lewis, however, it was a tough race to swallow. He could find solace in both his personal best and his new American record. But the fact remained that he had improved on his 9.93 in Rome a year before, yet finished even farther behind Ben. There were no credible alibis for a loss by thirteen hundredths.

Upon further analysis, the numbers for Lewis were even worse than they'd appeared. If you compared actual running times (by subtracting reaction times from finish times), Ben had improved by five hundredths in the last year, from 9.71 in Rome to 9.66 in Korea. Lewis, by contrast, ran five hundredths *slower* in Seoul, going from 9.74 to 9.79. He improved his final time only because he went from a poor reaction in Rome to a good one in Seoul. The Olympics showed that Ben had continued to expand his total energy envelope while Lewis had not.

With hindsight, it may be that Lewis's training concentrated too much on his start (his relative weak point before Rome) and too little on his last 40 metres, his great strength. To a degree, Carl had no choice. He *had* to improve early because Ben was getting so far in front that he could not possibly catch up. But he and his coach, Tom Tellez, may have overcompensated.

Leading up to Seoul, Lewis may have spent months to trim one hundredth off his start. The same effort might have gained him three or four hundredths in his finish. If I were his coach, I'd want to determine *where* Carl had reached his highest velocity: in races where he started more smoothly (and slowly), as at the Los Angeles Olympics, or where he started more explosively, as in Rome and Seoul? The answer would tell me which pattern I should build on. Lewis had shown in Rome that he was already capable of a 9.87 if he put together his best reaction time with his best running. If he could slice one more hundredth from each of his last five 10-metre segments (a realistic goal), he could get down to 9.82.

Of course, he *still* wouldn't have beaten Ben Johnson that day in South Korea.

Ben's race answered all the questions save one: How fast could he have gone if he had run all-out to the tape? In a post-race interview Ben noted that he "eased off the last two, three metres, or I'd have gone about 9.75. But I'm saving that for next year."

I believe his estimate was too conservative. The films showed that Ben had begun to ease off at the 80-metre mark, when he cut back on his arm drive. At that point he was nine hundredths ahead of his pace in Rome. If Ben had merely stayed *even* with his Rome pace from that point to the finish line, he would have run a 9.74, as compared to his Rome final time of 9.83. But it seems more probable that Ben would have continued to *improve* on his Rome pace from 80 to 100 metres, for two reasons. First, his training up to Seoul hinted that his speed endurance was better than ever before, which should have blunted or even reversed his late-race deceleration. Second, he entered those last 20 metres in Seoul at a higher velocity than in Rome—and therefore should have continued to run faster at each point of the deceleration curve.

If Ben had continued to better his Rome pace at the same rate he'd improved over the first 80 metres (that is, at about one hundredth per 10 metres), he would have shown a total improvement of ten hundredths, and therefore run a 9.72—twenty hundredths faster than Lewis, or eight feet better than anyone else at this distance in the history of the world.

And if Ben's last 20 metres had *exceeded* his rate of improvement over the first 80 (a possibility, since his finish in Rome was easily the weakest part of his race there), a 9.71 was conceivable, if not likely.

These calculations assume a relatively neutral racing environment: at sea level, with a legal tailwind of less than two metres per second. But what if Ben had run the same race in the thinner air of Mexico City, where Jim Hines set a world and Olympic record of 9.95 in 1968? The standard differential for 7,300 feet of altitude is eleven hundredths, but the higher the runner's speed, the larger the differential; air resistance becomes a greater factor when you're going faster, since you're pushing against more molecules over the same span of time. In Ben's case the differential might be twelve hundredths, dropping his projected time as low as 9.60—or thirty-five hundredths faster than Hines.

To take it a final step, consider that sprinters were hand-timed until the late 1960s, and that electronic measurements added at least twenty-four hundredths to their times. Had Ben run his projected 9.72 with hand-timing, he would have finished at 9.5—a full 13 metres ahead of Harold Abrahams (later made famous in *Chariots of Fire*) in the 1924 Olympics; 8 metres ahead of Jesse Owens in his 1936 triumph in Berlin; more than 5 metres ahead of the great Bob Hayes in 1964. In an anthropological micro-second, the 100-metre game had changed so much—with more potent drugs, improved training techniques, superior track surfaces and shoes—that it hardly was the same game at all.

Celebration

Ben was still decelerating when the time flashed on the electronic board high above the stands, three numbers that raised the crowd's roar once more, my own hoarse shout included: *9.79*. I knew the time was unofficial, but it wouldn't be more than a hundredth off. (In this case, the official videotape, which was checked within minutes of the event, would confirm the preliminary reading.) Ben had called his shot. It was the moment we'd been working toward for so long, and I felt a moment of pure euphoria—for the win, first and foremost. Nothing approached the importance of winning; Ben's new record seemed almost immaterial, something we'd done before and might well do again. But to win at the Olympics—that was what lit me up as I watched the race replay on the scoreboard, to an echo of cheers. The journalists around me knew who I was, but thoughtfully kept their distance. For those precious few seconds I was alone with the image of Ben crossing the line—an image that clung to my mind's eye long after the big screen had faded.

Out on the track the post-race rituals began. Ben jogged toward the stands and the waiting photographers. For a moment Carl Lewis stood alone and dejected past the finish line. He recovered enough to approach Ben from behind; he clutched at Ben's shoulder and twisted him around, and the two rivals awkwardly shook hands. The courtesy completed, Ben was lifted by Desai in a bear hug. He then grabbed a proffered Canadian flag for the obligatory victory lap— in this instance, a reluctant half-lap, since Ben was so exhausted that he could barely move.

I made my way down from the press section, shaking hands along the way. As I passed Russ Rogers, the Americans' sprint coach who had feuded so bitterly with Lewis, he offered his personal congratulations, *sotto voce*: "Thank you." I found Waldemar at the warm-up area, and we embraced. Our physio wanted to work on Ben's sore Achilles for the relays a week hence, and so we picked our way under the stands, to the gathering point for the athletes' procession to the medal ceremony. But there was no getting to Ben at that moment. He was ringed five and six deep by journalists, swallowed by pandemonium. I called out to him, but he couldn't see or hear me.

Thirty minutes after the race, with the medal ceremony about to begin, Ben and Linford Christie were still waiting for Lewis. After stating his intention to shower and change, Carl had disappeared. The officials decided they would present the medals without Lewis, and actually started the procession before Carl slipped into line en route.

After his record performance in Rome the year before, Ben had taken considerable flak for receiving his medal in a plain green sweatsuit. This time he re-emerged into the arena in his official team whites. Save for a pant leg that clung inside a sock, the picture was perfect.

Unlike Princess Anne, the president of South Korea, 70,000 others in the stands, and a billion more through television, I didn't see that medal ceremony, nor did I much care to. Suddenly I felt exhausted, almost immobile; as my adrenaline ebbed, I was left with a weary sense of relief. We'd had far more to lose than to gain here. At the end of 1987, Ben had been so far superior to all others that an Olympic win should never have been in doubt. Only a string of disasters had made for suspense—a weight I was glad to throw off. *Thank God it's over*, I thought.

The Royal Canadian Mounted Police escorted Ben back to the stands, to take a phone call from Prime Minister Brian Mulroney. (Mulroney: "My congratulations on behalf of all Canadians. You were just marvellous.... There is an explosion of joy here in Ottawa." Ben: "Thank you.") Then the RCMP led Ben and Waldemar through a maze of tunnels to the doping control room, and I went back outside to the track.

Minutes before Ben's race, Angella Issajenko had been eliminated from her 100-metre quarter-final in a lacklustre 11.27. I found her sitting against a wall on the far side of the warm-up area, quiet and disconsolate—it was the ultimate heartbreak in a career that had seen more than its share of disappointments. After an injury-riddled European campaign, Angella had trained superbly in Tokyo just two weeks before, running the equivalent of the high 10.80s. I thought she was headed for the low 10.80s—on track for an Olympic medal.

But instead of getting faster in Seoul, as Ben had, Angella got slower. She had inexplicably gained 10 pounds since leaving Canada at the end of August, despite the fact that she'd barely picked at the miserable Village fare. (When athletes go off steroids and into a clearance period, they *lose* weight.) Her recent practice times had been dull, and in her quarter-final she was obviously labouring. Once again, the big one had slipped away from her—just as it had in 1980, with the Olympic boycott; in 1983, when a sciatic nerve problem ruined her World Championships at Helsinki; in 1984, when she'd strained her hamstring just before the Los Angeles Olympics; in 1987, with her unlucky photo finish at the World Indoor Championships and her sluggish reaction in Rome. Now she was almost 30 years old, and her Olympic career was almost surely over.

There was little to say, and so we sat wordlessly on the grass. I thought about how Angella had held our sprint team together in the early years. Our younger runners—including Ben—obtained priceless experience because Angella had been such a big drawing card, and meet promoters were willing to accept our entire group if they could get her to run. Angella had worked as hard as a person can, done everything asked of her. But as my first world-class sprinter, she had also suffered from my on-the-job apprenticeship, and particularly from faulty drug protocols. (With hindsight, I believe Angella would have profited if we'd kept her on Anavar and Dianabol, rather than switching to Estragol.) I had done my best but Angella had deserved better; I felt lost in regret. Such is a track coach's lot. You can never be completely happy unless *all* your people win, and at this level that never happens.

As it developed, Angella could not have won the gold in Seoul, even with the race of her life. The following day, Florence Griffith Joyner would capture the 100-metre final, waving her taloned hands before the finish, in a wind-aided but still mind-boggling 10.54. (Flo-Jo's reaction time, at .131 seconds, was even better than Ben's.) Evelyn Ashford, the 31-year-old veteran, took the silver in 10.83—nine feet behind the winner. As far as the rest of the track world was concerned, Flo-Jo's performance could only be described as cataclysmic. When she'd run her world record 10.49 in the U.S. Olympic trials two months before in Indianapolis (breaking Ashford's forbidding four-year-old record by *twenty-seven* hundredths, or almost *three times* the advance Ben had made in Rome), no one had believed it. The consensus was that the clock had malfunctioned. Before the race at Seoul, the G.D.R.'s top sprint coaches, Hille and Tepper, told me they felt certain that no woman would run under 10.80.

I too was stunned by Flo-Jo's achievement. Through 1987, her 100-metre career had been unremarkable. She hadn't significantly improved over the previous four years; Angella, among others, had beaten her consistently during that period. (Going into the 1988 season, in fact, Flo-Jo wasn't even ranked among the top 10 women in the world in the 100; *Track & Field News* rated her only seventh among the Americans in that event.) At the relatively advanced age of 28, Flo-Jo appeared most unlikely to leapfrog to the head of the class; for her to do so would have defied all precedent.

Yet leap she did. In one year she improved by an inconceivable forty-seven hundredths in the 100 and by sixty-two hundredths in the 200, blazing the latter in 21.34 seconds in her gold-medal run in the Olympics—*close to four tenths faster* than the old world record. Flo-Jo's new records warped the historical performance curves, the statistical projections of future records based on past performances. Her times had arrived more than 50 years ahead of schedule.

Shortly after the 100-metre final, according to Pete Axthelm in *Newsweek*, as the media gathered to ask Flo-Jo how she had run so fast, silver medallist Evelyn Ashford turned to her and said, "Why don't you tell them, Florence?" The snide arrow struck its mark. "When Evelyn broke a world record, I said it was an outstanding performance," an indignant Flo-Jo protested. "Now, in essence, she's accusing me of using drugs."

As often occurs after a race and the rigorous, dehydrating warm-ups that must precede it, Ben had a hard time producing a urine sample and was stalled in doping control for more than an hour after the race. In the meantime, the media heard from Lewis. For all his surface cool, it must have been an excruciating time for Carl, a day that struck at the core of his identity. In Rome he'd run a sea-level record and had been wiped out. In Seoul he'd done even better— and found himself finishing even farther behind. The strain began to show within seconds of Carl's post-race handshake with Ben. When a television interviewer asked about Ben's performance, Lewis said, "He must have really caught a flyer [out of the blocks], just like in Rome"—as if to insist that Ben had won the race at the start, against the reality that all had witnessed.

Minutes later, in the press room (a sunless, airless area under the stands that was flimsily partitioned by canvas flaps), Lewis ascended to his place behind a raised, cafeteria-style table. He began to sit behind the gold medallist's microphone—force of habit, perhaps—before moving to the silver medallist's chair. After a sound check, he asked an official to turn up his volume. Finally satisfied, he accepted questions from among two hundred seated reporters. Lewis would offer no alibis this time. Instead he would attempt to minimize what had happened on the track. Rivalry— what rivalry?

"We just go out to perform. That's what the Olympic Games are all about—performance. People come here to run their best and that's how it is," Carl said.

"My objective was to run a personal best and do the best I can. I did both those things, so that's why I'm happy with the way I ran."

After ducking repeated requests for comment on Ben's race, Lewis finally became exasperated, and blurted out: "He ran a great race, obviously, because he had a great time."

Long after Lewis had left the news conference, Ben remained stuck in doping control. "He's had two beers but nothing's happening," a Canadian official reported. "Mr. Ben Johnson is in doping [control] and he will be here in five minutes," a South Korean functionary announced every twenty minutes. The media people, as depicted in the Toronto *Globe and Mail*, were getting restless.

"Listen, Mr. Five Minutes, let's get him out here, we've got deadlines," an American writer yelled.

"He's gotta *pee*," a Canadian reporter shouted back. "Can you always pee when you want?"

When Ben finally appeared, nearly two hours after the race, he was decidedly relaxed. As I sat down beside him on the dais, he turned to me and confided, "I'm shit-faced." He'd needed *ten* beers to produce the required sample, and the ensuing scene was worthy of Fellini. Ben offered his stock post-race comments—"I was prepared"; "I did the same thing in Rome"—but none of his answers bore any relation to the questions posed to him. Since the reporters weren't miked and the room was large, only the individual questioner knew that Ben wasn't responding; the rest of them scribbled dutifully in their notebooks. At that, Ben's remarks rang truer than those of the man who had preceded him. His pride showed through: "I'd like to say my name is Benjamin Sinclair Johnson, Jr., and this world record will last 50 years, maybe 100." Then he went to the heart of the matter.

"The important thing," Ben said, "was to beat Carl."

The rewards of Ben's achievement in Seoul were more than emotional. Many of Ben's endorsement contracts (including his deal with Diadora) featured separate bonus clauses for Olympic gold medals *and* for world records; the total dividend would exceed $300,000. Larry Heidebrecht predicted that Ben would at least double his income in the coming year, beginning with an October 8th showdown with Lewis in Tokyo that would net Ben $500,000. In addition, Nissan had offered to sponsor the Optimists, pending Ben's winning the gold medal, with a seven-figure, multi-year contract. In the first year alone, Nissan would pay the team several times what we'd been receiving from Mazda. The lion's share of the contract would go to Ben, but there would be enough left over to recompense Astaphan and Waldemar (both of whom had been underpaid for years), and to help support athletes like Angella and Mark who were almost totally dependent on appearance fees. For the first time, it looked like my top people would be able to train without worrying about money. After years of scrounging for a few extra dollars to hold my program together, I could now turn my full attention to what I enjoyed most—coaching.

Then again, I knew that my coaching career was in its twilight, if only because I'd come to focus on mature athletes and had left the younger ones to my assistants. Within a few years, I assumed that I would become more of a consultant, like Gerard Mach. In the meantime, I felt certain, Ben Johnson and I would have many opportunities to lower his record time still further. Ben had improved steadily since he started, by at least six hundredths a year, and had yet to begin levelling off. It was unlikely that his progress would halt abruptly. It seemed more probable that he would improve at least another two or three hundredths the next year (and perhaps another one or two the year after that) before hitting the wall. That meant that we might take the record down into the 9.60s, a terrain that no one had dreamed of.

I had no way of knowing that Seoul would represent our last best chance together—or that less than two days after we'd reached the summit, we would tumble down at a speed to dizzy even the world's fastest human.

Inquiry

The days after the Olympic final passed in fast-forward. The first news of Ben's positive "A" sample, our meeting with Beckett and Donike, the appeal pressed by Dick Pound, our hurried exits from Seoul—all of it raced by. But as the days blurred into weeks, and the media's obsession with our story gradually abated, the pace slowed. It was mostly a time for reflection and transition, for plotting legal strategies for the hearings to come, for adjusting to my new life outside track. It was a dark period, clouded by disappointment. I couldn't help thinking of how I'd thrown my whole life into coaching, until I'd reached the very top, only to lose it all—my career, my reputation, even my day-to-day routines.

Finally, five months after Ben's suspension, the Dubin Inquiry (known officially as the Commission of Inquiry into the Use of Drugs and Banned Practices Intended to Increase Athletic Performance) commenced proceedings in Toronto in February 1989. Appointed by the Mulroney government, Ontario's associate chief justice, Charles Dubin, would be the sole presiding official. He had a sweeping mandate, as announced by then-sport minister Jean Charest, to "restore the integrity of sport in Canada." To that end, Dubin could subpoena any coach, athlete, or official in Canada to testify. He also had the power to recommend criminal charges if he deemed them necessary.

As I saw it, I could only gain by providing the Inquiry with the fullest and most detailed truth. I had lost my career and my athletes. I'd been branded a cheat, a Svengali, and even (by the more imaginative commentators) a pusher of drugs to children. I'd been portrayed as a coach who took short cuts because he couldn't succeed in any other way. The Olympic gold medal we'd worked so hard for 12 years to attain now belonged to our most bitter rival; the world record Ben had set in Rome would soon be washed away as well. All of our work together was discredited.

I knew that my testimony would seal my fate within the industry. In a sport steeped in hypocrisy, there is no place for a candid man. But while my career was a dead issue, I thought I might still salvage my reputation and those of my athletes. Once people were made aware of the larger environment which framed my actions, I thought that they might lay aside the cardboard villain who bore my name after Seoul.

There was more at stake, of course, than my personal honour. In giving my testimony, I hoped that others would be induced to follow my lead. If every coach and athlete told the truth about drug use, it would force a public re-evaluation of sport—of what our society sought from the arena, and what practices it was prepared to accept. However painful that process might be, it would certainly improve the current environment in track and field, a realm of cynical fans, sanctimonious administrators, and backstabbing superstars, where what you do (or take) matters less than your ability to hide it.

After 29 hours of testimony, I was exhausted but relieved. Once you've decided to tell *everything*, most of the pressure dissolves. With nothing to hide, I could not slip up or contradict myself. I've always had a good memory (which helped me sift through the welter of dates, running times, and drug protocols I needed to summon up), but it's easier to remember the unvarnished truth—it's the lies that tax us most.

In the thousands of pages of sworn testimony that succeeded my own, the Inquiry laid to rest any lingering illusions as to the extent of doping in track and field. A number of witnesses, called as experts or inside observers, corroborated my basic premise: that you could not expect to win without drugs against the sport's elite. Dr. Robert Kerr outlined the steroid protocols used throughout the world, and testified that he had prescribed steroids for 20 U.S. medallists at the 1984 Olympics. Bill Crothers, a 1964 Olympic silver medallist and Toronto pharmacist, estimated that six of the eight finalists in the 100 metres at Seoul were using anabolic steroids. Several throwers, including Bishop Dolegiewicz, asserted that steroids were considered essential to get within three metres of the world shot-put record. And West German sportscaster Bernd Heller testified to Manfred Donike's admission that 80 percent of the male track and field athletes at Seoul had "positive" endocrine profiles—the testing tool used to trap Ben Johnson, but which has yet to be applied against anyone else.

For other, more vulnerable witnesses (and most obviously for my athletes), the sport's pervasive hypocrisy put them between a rock and the hardest of places. The worst dilemma belonged to Ben. He had two choices, neither of them palatable. He could deny his drug use and attempt to limit the sanctions against him, a tactic which would alienate the Canadian public. Or he could admit to using steroids at the cost of severe penalties from the IAAF.

Ben had stonewalled until emerging evidence made it untenable. Allowed to take the stand last among the Optimist principals, Ben could not overcome the cumulative weight of prior testimony—by me, Angella, Astaphan (who brought along a taped phone conversation with Ben in which steroids were openly discussed), and several other Mazda athletes. Once on the stand, he switched to admission, apology, and all the usual platitudes. He'd been wrong to take drugs, Ben now maintained: "I want to say drugs can't make you run faster." With the obligatory admonition to the nation's youth—"Don't take drugs. I've been there"—Ben offered less a defence than a *mea culpa*.

The testimony of IAAF lab directors and officials—notably that of Manfred Donike of Cologne and Arne Ljungqvist of Sweden (the IAAF vice-president and chairman of both its Medical Committee and Doping Commission)—told much about the vagaries of drug-testing procedures. In his recollection of the two reported testosterone positives at the 1983 World Championships in Helsinki, Donike testified that the two ratios involved were indeed above the permitted 6:1, but said that no action had been taken because the urine samples were judged "too dilute."

During his turn on the stand, Ljungqvist first said that he "couldn't remember" the cases in question. After his memory was refreshed by a copy of a newspaper story about one of the positives, Ljungqvist proceeded to disagree with Donike's testimony, maintaining that the two ratios were *below* 6:1. (This puzzled some observers, since a ratio within the allowable limit would not ordinarily come to the attention of lab personnel in the first place.)

Under cross-examination, Donike also admitted that he had been able to identify Ben's urine sample from the 1988 Zurich *Weltklasse* (with the aid of IAAF headquarters in London) *months after that meet*, and had proceeded to re-test the specimen. The Zurich sample came up negative a second time, Donike confirmed.

Once again, Ben had been singled out. If the coded name lists remained on file, officials could have used them to go after every other person found to have a positive endocrine profile at the Seoul Olympics, as well as at prior meets. Instead, they sat on these explosive data—findings which could have led to the suspension of untold numbers of athletes.

Donike's testimony raised other disturbing possibilities. If the name lists were available indefinitely, and—as acknowledged on the stand by Robert Dugal, head of the IOC-accredited laboratory in Montreal—extraordinary measures could be taken to find banned substances in the samples of known competitors, what was there to prevent the IAAF from compiling information on a given athlete who was considered troublesome? What if it were finally deemed convenient for that athlete to be expelled from the sport? If there was no integrity in this system's confidentiality, could we assume integrity in its results?

The second theme to emerge at the Dubin Inquiry was the IAAF's impotence in compelling its member federations to enforce its anti-doping policies. "The IAAF is not a police force," Ljungqvist told the inquiry. During a recent BBC telecast, he was echoed by John Holt of the IAAF: "We've always said we haven't got an international police force. We don't actually go to individual athletes, we always go to [the] national federations."

In other words, the IAAF relies on an honour system in an arena where international prestige and millions of dollars are at issue. The consequences of that system were laid bare by Ljungqvist on the witness stand. Had the IAAF investigated published comments by Hans-Jürgen Noczenski, a former high official of the East German Olympic Committee, that the G.D.R. systematically administered steroids to its international athletes? (The East Germans were pre-tested at home before international competitions to ensure that steroid users would test negatively after the meets, Noczenski had told *Das Bild*, a West German newspaper. "Those that were clean were allowed to compete. Those that weren't were told to say that they were injured.") Had the IAAF looked into the claim made by *Zmena*, the Communist party youth magazine, that the Soviets have systematically doped their athletes for years? Had the organization checked out two testosterone positives (as confirmed by the director of the UCLA medical lab) at the U.S.A. Mobil Indoor Track and Field Championships in February 1989, which were later overturned by The Athletics Congress? In each case, Ljungqvist acknowledged that nothing had been done. In reference to East Germany, he passed off Noczenski's public charges as "innuendo and rumour."

The only acceptable forum for such allegations, Ljungqvist added, would be at a hearing convened by either the IAAF or by the national federation involved. Here was a classic Catch-22: The IAAF has never convened such a hearing, while its member feder-ations could hardly be expected to sink their own ships. Without a hearing, the officials aver, there is no admissible evidence. Without admissible evidence, there can be no sanctions.

It was little wonder when an exasperated Bob Armstrong, the Dubin Inquiry's tireless chief counsel, concluded that "the last 16 years of competition testing has been largely a waste of time and money."

The IAAF's meek deference to its more powerful national constituents (and particularly the Big Three—the United States, the Soviet Union, and East Germany) stood in pointed contrast to its draconian treatment of Canada. The greater outrage is that our own Ontario Track and Field Association laid the foundation for this double standard. In March 1989, immediately after Angella Issajenko's testimony followed my own, the OTFA banned me from coaching for five years, and passed a resolution to strip all provincial records from any athletes who acknowledged taking steroids. This move set off a testy exchange between Commissioner Charles Dubin and Rolf Lund, the OTFA president who testified later that spring.

The OTFA's resolution, Dubin lectured, "told anybody who would come forth...that if they admitted their use of steroids, they'd be penalized.... You were discouraging people from coming forward and telling the truth.... Why did that have to be done then?"

The undeniable effect of the OTFA's sanction was to protect the rest of its coaches and athletes, even as the Mazda group was drawn and quartered. As long as my sprinters could be held up as exceptions to a virtuous rule, the OTFA's public support and revenues would not be imperilled. For Lund and his cohorts, the narrower the Inquiry's scope, the better.

After the OTFA made it clear that athletes would be punished for telling the truth, the IAAF followed suit. Shortly after the Inquiry convened, August Kirsch, an IAAF council member from West Germany, stated that Ben's 9.83 in Rome would stand as the 100-metre world record, since Ben had passed the drug test there. "The rules on this matter are clear," Kirsch said. "There is nothing we can do about that." But Kirsch had underestimated the creativity of IAAF president Primo Nebiolo. On September 4, 1989, at a delegates' session in Barcelona described by Jean-Guy Ouellette as "a real zoo," Nebiolo rammed through a rule to nullify world records by athletes who confessed to drug use under oath. It would not matter whether the athletes took or passed a drug test at the meet in question. The admission alone would trigger the penalty.

The new sanction was blatantly selective, most of all in its retroactivity. My athletes had been the only active competitors forced to testify candidly about their drug use, since they were the only ones with prior evidence against them: my testimony. It was no coincidence that *every other active athlete* called by Dubin would deny using drugs. Their testimony was safe; there was no one to contradict them.

The Inquiry's selectivity was heightened by its decision to focus exclusively on two sports, weightlifting and track and field. Other sports where doping is *known* to be rampant worldwide, including cycling, swimming and rowing, were ignored.

Four world records were struck down retroactively by the Barcelona vote: Ben's 9.83 in the 100 metres in Rome, his 6.41 in the 60, and his 5.55 in the 50, and Angella Issajenko's 6.06 in the 50. It was hard to say who had been more abused. Ben's record in the 100 passed to Carl Lewis, even though Ben had tested negative at Rome—the only standard for validating a winning or record performance in more than 20 years of drug testing. Angella's mark passed to Marita Koch of the steroid-saturated G.D.R., who had not even been tested when her now-recognized record was set.

Ben and Angella could have kept their records under the Barcelona rule—but only if they had previously perjured themselves by disclaiming their use of steroids when under oath at the Dubin Inquiry. The IAAF had sent out a peremptory warning to other athletes, and particularly to the Eastern Europeans who were leaving their countries in droves for the West: Tell the truth at your peril. As IOC vice-president Richard Pound noted, "The problem of drugs in sports is pretty complicated; it's not going to be solved by this kind of a ruling.... This really enforces a code of silence."

In his questioning of Ljungqvist, Armstrong declared that the Barcelona rule was "a backward step" in the anti-doping war, since it could only encourage lying, cheating, and the suppression of valuable information. "The effect of that rule," Armstrong said, "could well be to send out a message around the world: 'Simply keep your mouth shut and continue to do what you've always done—deny, deny, deny, and there will be no problem.' "

Ljungvist had to concede Armstrong's point, but maintained that nothing had been lost, since athletes seldom volunteer the truth anyway. Shortly thereafter, Ljungkvist hurried off to catch a plane. For the IAAF, life would go on—with business as usual.

Of all that I heard at the Dubin Inquiry, one revelation was particularly distressing. It emerged when Glen Bogue, the CTFA's manager of athlete services, testified that he first became aware of possible drug use within our sprint group in 1985. Bogue was relying on more than third-hand rumours. According to his testimony, he had an inside source: Desai Williams, who'd remained friendly with Ben and his other old teammates after leaving the group in 1983. According to Bogue, Desai called him to offer specific information about banned substances among my athletes—and in particular about Ben's use of steroids, which Desai said he feared might endanger Ben's health.

The discussion didn't stop there. During the same phone call, Bogue testified, Desai agreed to let Bogue know when the CTFA might successfully surprise Ben with a random test. Desai's name would not be disclosed in the operation, Bogue assured him. This was truly a sordid tale—a case of the second-fastest man in Canada, who would later acknowledge his own use of steroids, informing on the one countryman who could beat him. Although Desai disputed the details of Bogue's testimony, Dubin concluded in his report that Bogue "accurately recounted the substance of the conversation." Moreover, the Commissioner drily added, "I do not think it was Mr. Johnson's health that Mr. Williams was concerned about since, if it were, a private chat with Mr. Johnson would have been the appropriate means of dealing with it."

In July 1990—15 months after my testimony concluded, nearly two years after Seoul—Commissioner Dubin submitted his report. For myself, it amounted to a semi-vindication. Dubin condemned my use of steroids as a training tool, and recommended that my salary from Sport Canada be severed, a foregone conclusion. At the same time, the Commissioner noted, "It was conceded by all witnesses that Mr. Francis was devoted to his athletes to the point where no sacrifice by him in favour of his group was too much to make." Dubin also tallied several mitigating factors in any appeal I might make of my indefinite suspension by the CTFA: my "full co-operation" with the Commission; my contribution to the sport; and "the care and development of [my] athletes apart from [my] involvement with drugs."

Ben came off less well. Referring to the commercialized environment of international track, "in which winning was the only measure of success and the means of financial reward," Dubin allowed that he could "understand the circumstances that led Mr. Johnson to use performance-enhancing substances. I cannot understand how, after his return from Seoul...he would allow himself to be a party to an orchestrated plan he knew would mislead the Canadian public and the international sporting community into believing he had never used performance-enhancing drugs."

Dubin noted, however, that Ben's eligibility to compete at the end of his two-year suspension must be decided by the CTFA— which had already made clear that it would welcome Ben back. And he slammed the IAAF's retroactive stripping of Ben's and Angella's world records as violating "every principle of natural justice and fairness." In addition, the Commissioner wrote, the IAAF's Barcelona rule (under which athletes can be found guilty of doping through their own admissions, even if they have tested negative at the meet or meets in question) would "encourage the continuation of the conspiracy of silence" and "discourage athletes who would otherwise have been willing to aid in cleaning up the sport from coming forward....

"In view of the testimony before this Commission, there is no guarantee that the world records that replaced those which were stripped are any less tainted, or that all the records still standing were made by drug-free athletes."

Dubin generally accepted the picture of international track—and of pervasive drug use—that I'd painted on the witness stand: "As shocking as Mr. Francis's evidence initially appeared when he testified before this Inquiry, much of what he said was supported by many other witnesses. Also, disclosures made subsequent to his testimony have tended to provide further confirmation."

More specifically, the Commissioner took a hard line toward the sport's governing bodies, from the IOC to the CTFA, whose reluctance to enforce random testing has laid bare their pretences of "clean" competition. In what amounted to a vote of no confidence in the dope busters, he endorsed the establishment of a new, "independent world doping control agency."

Dubin acknowledged that drug use was "so prevalent" that it was "worth considering whether, at present, success in international competition is still a worthy objective." He also recommended that carding subsidies be tied to "domestic standards" rather than international ones—an indirect admission that Canadians could no longer be expected to keep up with the world's elite. But Dubin stopped short of pushing his findings to their logical conclusion: that a dope-free Canadian program cannot succeed in the drug-drenched milieu of international track.

The unassailable fact is that a "pure" Canadian team will win far more plaudits than medals at the Olympics and other major international meets. It is simply not enough for a Canadian Olympic Association to "urge" the IOC to ban national organizations lacking an effective doping-control policy, as Dubin suggested, nor for the CTFA to follow suit with the IAAF. Such urgings from a minor player will mean little against the vast power and money invested in the status quo.

As columnist Robert Payne wrote in *The Toronto Sun*:

"If I read the Dubin recommendations clearly, Canada's Olympic hopes will soon rest on the Miss Congeniality Award. We may as well declare ourselves a medal-free nation, at least in sports where steroids are swallowed as readily as Gatorade.... The gaping flaw in

Dubin's recommendations is that they finger only Canadians. For Americans, Brits, Germans, et al., it will be business as usual.

"To be fair, Mr. Justice Dubin has recommended that Canada confine its international competition to nations equally prepared to drug-bust. But whom? Liechtenstein?"

While I was generally pleased by Dubin's report, I was at least as gratified by an earlier judgement, a week after my testimony had concluded. I was walking down University Avenue in Toronto when a young man in an old Chevrolet jammed on his brakes, jumped out of his car, and walked straight up to me. I'd never seen him before and didn't know what to expect at first, but the man's smile disarmed me. "Good job, Charlie," he said. He shook my hand, got back in his car, and drove off. I never saw him again, but I'll never forget him. Track coaches tend to keep a low profile, unto invisibility. Through all my years as a sprint coach, no one had ever recognized me on the street. I'd gained my fame only after the fall.

Eighty Nanograms
in South Korea

To this day, I cannot say for certain why Ben Johnson tested positive in Seoul. I can offer only a mixed bag of hypotheses—some of them contradictory, others mutually supporting, none of them airtight—which might begin to suggest how the biggest scandal in Olympic history came to pass.

Ben was sabotaged. Although this idea has been dismissed by both Commissioner Charles Dubin and the IOC, I believe it is possible that Ben's fatal positive in Seoul was the result of tampering before the test. A spiked drink wouldn't have affected Ben's endocrine profile, the dubious tool that did us in. But the only pretext for examining that profile was Ben's positive for stanozolol—a result which *could* have been induced by a tainted drink after the race. (As the IOC's Arnold Beckett had confirmed to me during Ben's preliminary hearing, stanozolol begins to metabolize inside the body within 45 minutes to one hour.) If security in the doping control room was indeed compromised, as alleged by several individuals present at that time (including Don Wilson, the Royal Canadian Mounted Police officer), then the IOC Medical Commission's case against Ben was constructed on shaky ground.

In a variant of this scenario, someone might have used stanozolol to adulterate the anti-inflammatory rub used daily by Waldemar throughout our stay at Seoul. (The rub also contained dimethyl-sulfoxide, or DMSO, a carrier agent which would help transmit the anti-inflammatory—and any steroid present—through the skin and into the bloodstream.) Tainting the rub would have been easier and less risky than foul play in the testing room, since it would require only brief access to Waldemar's trainer's bag at any time after we left Vancouver on September 6th. While this theory received short shrift from the experts, it is pertinent to note that topical steroids—chiefly Andractim Gel, a brand of dihydrotestosterone manufactured in Belgium—are commonly rubbed through the skin in Europe.

My concerns about sabotage were magnified after Seoul by a conversation with Anne-Lise Hammer, the Norwegian journalist, regarding some suspicious business between a prominent athlete and a meet official in Sweden in 1987. The official reportedly asked the athlete to procure some Stromba (stanozolol) tablets on my behalf for Ben—a ridiculous idea at a time when we were pointing toward a world record through a series of tested meets. It occurred to me that someone might have been trying to set us up for a debacle in Rome three weeks later—to establish a steroid trail that would have led to us had Ben tested positive at the World Championships.

Finally, there remains the question of the American stranger who hovered over Ben during his 90 fateful minutes in the doping control room after the 100-metre final at Seoul. The IOC officials in charge denied ever seeing such a person. While Commissioner Dubin acknowledged the stranger's existence, his commission failed to establish the person's identity, leaving Dubin to conclude that there "was no evidence...that this stranger had administered any drug to Mr. Johnson."

Almost two years after Seoul, in June of 1990, new light on this matter was shed by a most unlikely source: Carl Lewis. In Lewis's *Inside Track*, Carl identifies the mystery man as André Jackson, an old friend who stayed with Lewis's family in Seoul. The book even includes two photographs of Jackson sitting next to Ben in doping control—and in close proximity to a can of beer Ben was drinking. According to *Inside Track*, Jackson originally entered the area out of curiosity, but decided to stick around to make sure that Waldemar "did not give Ben anything more than a rubdown before Ben urinated into his drug-test bottle.... He had heard me and others on the track circuit talk about Ben doing drugs, and he was suspicious...."

I have no evidence that André Jackson was in any way responsible for Ben's positive at Seoul, but the fact remains that he has yet to be officially questioned about his unauthorized presence in the doping control room.

Ben was freelancing. I knew that Ben had a home supply of oral stanozolol, or Winstrol, which he'd received from Dr. Astaphan. As far as I knew, he'd last used the pills in the spring of 1987. Although I couldn't be sure what he'd been taking during his stay with Astaphan in St. Kitts in May and June of 1988 (or what he might have done on his own that summer), any problem would have surfaced in his test at Zurich, six weeks before the Olympic final. (The Zurich test was re-evaluated by Donike after Seoul, and confirmed as negative.)

In any case, it seemed unlikely that the Winstrol tablets had caused Ben's positive. If Ben had taken them less than five days before his final (the clearance time suggested by Arnold Beckett), the only possible effect would be detrimental—a retention of fluid which would tighten Ben's muscles. But Waldemar found no such stiffness in Seoul, and Ben's form through his final practices—not to mention his 9.79—precluded any impairment.

The question of Ben's freelancing surfaced again at the Dubin Inquiry, after his attorney introduced evidence that Ben had developed gynecomastia (the formation of discernible breast tissue in the male) in October 1987. But while gynecomastia is an occasional side effect of steroid use, it would be unlikely to stem from either stanozolol or furazabol, since these particular substances do little to *aromatize*, or convert androgens to estrogens within the body. There appeared to be three possible causes of Ben's condition:

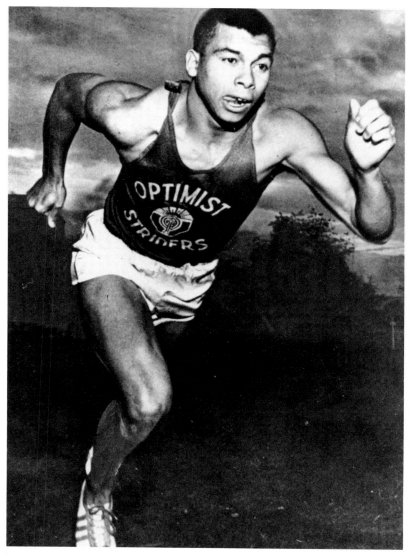

Harry Jerome was the fastest man in Canada in the 1960s—a world record-holder who was celebrated abroad but slighted at home. (British Columbia Sports Hall of Fame Archives)

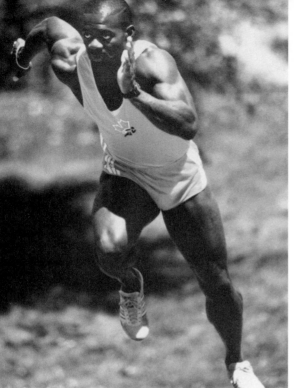

Ben displays ideal form during start practice at York University in 1987. His body forms a straight line from his neck to his left heel—the better to put all of Ben's power to work. (Gray Mortimore/Allsport)

Preparing for our national championships in July 1987, I help Angella Issajenko stretch. Angella went on to win both the 100 and 200 metres, as usual; over a 10-year span, she placed first in all 17 of the national sprint titles she contested. (Toronto Sun)

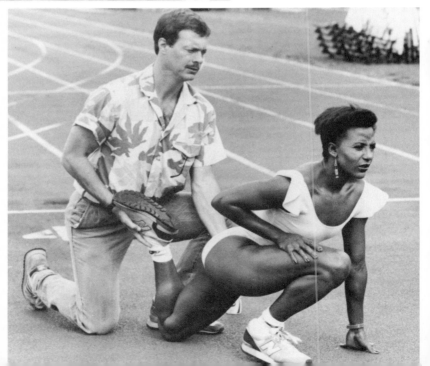

Ben leaps from the starting blocks at the World Championships in Rome in August 1987, on his way to a world-record time of 9.83 seconds. His superior reaction time in this race—.129 seconds—would account for two-thirds of his final margin over Carl Lewis. (A. G. Giumanni/ Foto ANSA)

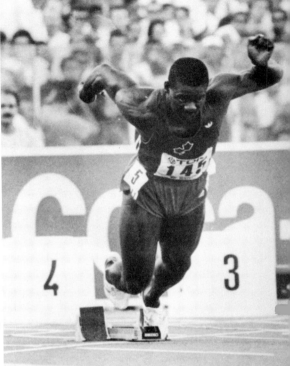

By the 20-metre mark in Rome, Ben has already sprinted to daylight from the field. Note the extension of Ben's rear leg and the vertical line of his torso; while his opponents remain in transition from their starting phase, Ben is in full running stride. (Antonio Beltrami)

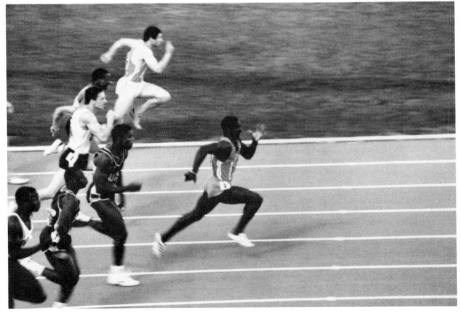

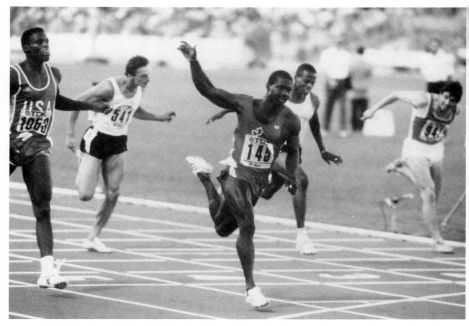

At the finish in Rome, Ben defeats Carl Lewis by a full tenth of a second, a margin of more than three feet. (Tony Duffy/Allsport)

Ben and I consult at practice in July 1988, shortly after our reconciliation, and just two months before the Olympics. (Gary Hershorn/Reuter)

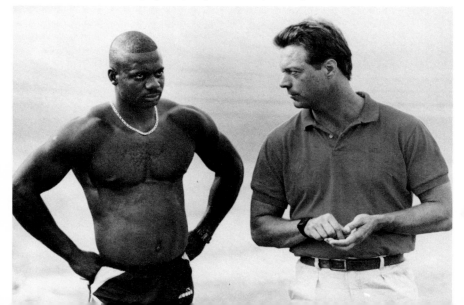

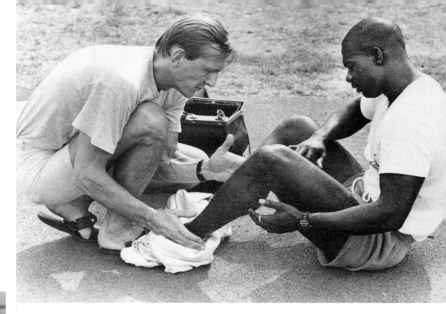

Waldemar Matuszewski, the best physiotherapist in the world, rubs down those million-dollar legs. (Gary Hershorn/Reuter)

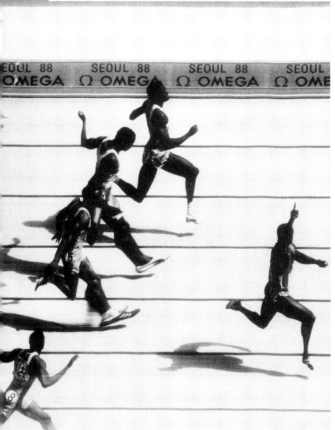

This official Swiss Timing photo captures Ben hitting the finish line at Seoul in a world-record 9.79 seconds, despite his raising his right arm—in a drastic deceleration—to celebrate the gold medal. Ben is glaring squarely at his old rival, Carl Lewis, who responds with a dour look of his own. (AP)

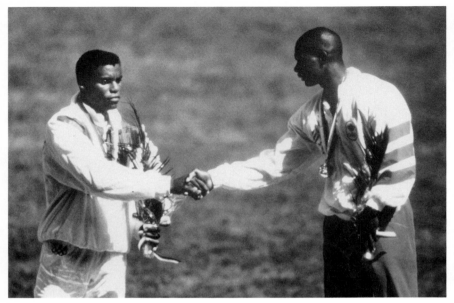

On the Olympic victory stand, a dejected Carl Lewis offers his hand to the world's fastest human. (Peter Read Miller/Sports Illustrated)

Fresh from victory at Seoul, Ben proceeds to his fateful drug test. (Gary Hershorn/Reuter)

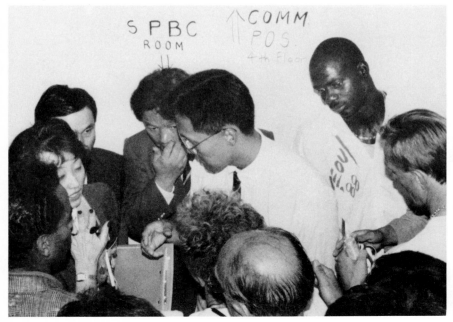

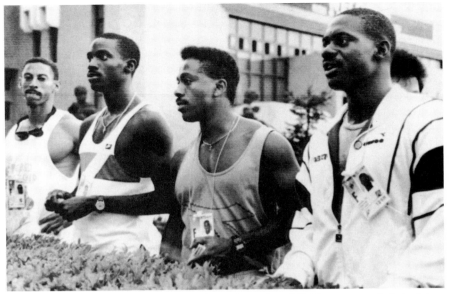

Four prominent members of Canada's Olympic track and field team tour their training facilities shortly after arriving in Seoul in September 1988. From left, they are Mark McCoy, the quiet hurdler with sprinter's speed; Anton Skerritt, Canada's 400-metre record-holder, who was coached by my old mentor, Percy Duncan; Desai Williams, my first big talent; and Ben Johnson, a week before his 100-metre final. (Reuter)

Tightly surrounded by security guards, Ben makes his way through Kimpo Airport for his flight back to Toronto. (Ronald C. Modra/Sports Illustrated)

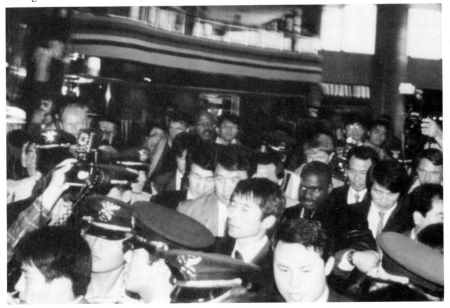

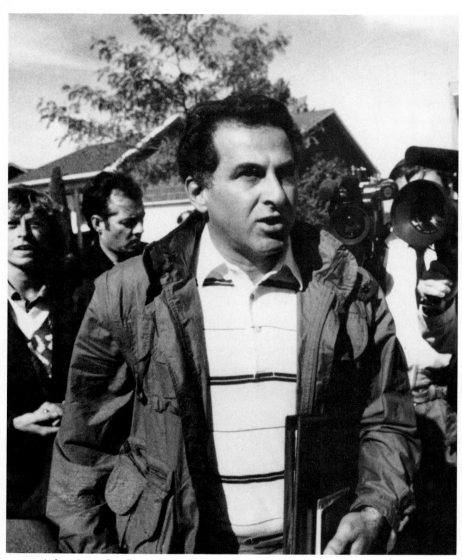

A few days after Ben's Olympic disqualification, Dr. Jamie Astaphan runs a media gauntlet to get to Ben's house in suburban Toronto. (Fred Lum/Globe and Mail)

He was experiencing a delayed onset of adolescent gynecomastia, which can occur without drugs; he was getting a late "rebound" from natural testosterone in response to his last stanozolol injections four months before; or he was taking an aromatizing steroid, such as testosterone or Anadrol-50, without my knowledge.

Dr. Astaphan blundered. This theory was floated by Gary Lubin, a Toronto coach. According to Lubin, Astaphan informed him that he'd injected Ben with "a little something extra" four days before Ben's final, and once again four hours before the race. This was preposterous. No experienced doctor would jeopardize a sprinter's performance by injecting an anabolic steroid so close to race time—whether with the untestable furazabol (which we believed our athletes were getting) or the testable stanozolol (the drug that Astaphan actually provided). In addition, Ben was on the warm-up track four hours before his race. I know, because I was with him—and I know that Astaphan was not.

Lubin's account aside, the conventional wisdom has targeted Ben's three steroid injections in August 1988 as a desperate lapse in judgement by Astaphan and myself. Dubin endorsed this analysis in his report: "There had been a dramatic deterioration in [Ben's] performance, and I think they panicked.... To embark on a steroid program so close to a competition was risky and they knew it." In fact, there was nothing unusual about the August injections. The last of them was administered 26 days before the 100-metre final in Seoul—well beyond the minimum safety margin we thought we needed. Ben had tested negative on numerous occasions with a clearance time of 26 days or less. Our steroid protocol that summer was routine.

In retrospect, however, there *was* a disquieting aspect to Astaphan's preparations before the race in Seoul. Before we left Toronto that August, he arranged for our sprinters to receive treatment on a diapulse machine—something he'd never done before—to help remove the steroids from their systems. In both Toronto and Tokyo (where we stopped for a preliminary meet in early September), Astaphan administered a diuretic called Moduret. While the doctor had intermittently given diuretics to our athletes in the past to prevent weight gain, I noticed that he was doubling the normal dose—perhaps as an additional measure to flush steroids from the sprinters' bodies. At the time I attributed Astaphan's anxiety to the slight chance that we might be tested at the Tokyo meet, a worry that proved unfounded. That failed to explain, however, why the doctor provided bottles of honey and vinegar—a reputed masking agent—for Ben and Desai to drink on the day of the 100-metre final in Seoul. (Ben would testify that he never drank it.) I'd never known Astaphan to resort to this last-minute tactic before. Taken together, his actions suggest that Ben may have taken an additional steroid dose *after* August 28th—either from the doctor or on his own.

The fat theory. After Ben's hamstring injuries forced him to curtail his speed drills and to do extra weightlifting to compensate, he was ten pounds over his racing weight two months before Seoul. As he lost that weight, traces of stanozolol, stored in his fat tissue from several weeks before, might have spurted into his system shortly before he was tested. But this theory contains several holes. To begin with, Ben remained extremely lean even at his heaviest; most of his weight gain was in muscle. Further, the lab found 80 nanograms (parts per billion) of stanozolol metabolites in Ben's urine sample—16 times greater than the minimum for a positive test, and far more than would be expected under this scenario. Subsequent testing also showed *undifferentiated* stanozolol—that is, pure steroid not yet converted into its primary metabolites. Since the body breaks down stanozolol within a range of one hour (after oral ingestion) to a few days (after an injection), the lab analysis indicates a close pre-race administration.

The labs improved their collection procedures. Dope-testing technologies are continually advancing. A new procedure might have enabled the lab to trace stanozolol metabolites beyond the accepted

14-day clearance time. (More recent advances have reportedly enabled the tracking of stanozolol *up to 22 weeks* after the last dose.) If this were the reason for Ben's positive, however, it would suggest that other Olympic medallists would have been snared as well. Under various brand names (oral Stromba and injectable Strombaject in Europe, oral Winstrol and injectable Winstrol-V in the U.S.), stanozolol had become the world-class sprinter's steroid of choice by 1988. It was used systematically in East Germany and extensively in West Germany, Britain, Italy, and the Soviet Union. If Ben tested positive because of improved collection techniques alone, *many* other athletes should also have been caught.

Beyond the perplexing fact of Ben's positive, there is a larger mystery: Why was the test result allowed to surface to the attention of the press and public? The powers that be, after all, have a vested interest in how the tests come out. They need to catch a few lesser lights now and then, to lend credibility to their operations. But if too many people—or even one or two big stars—test positive, it could endanger the sport's future, not to mention lab contracts and revenues. Damage control at international meets would not be without precedent. Specimens can become "too dilute"; results can be "interpreted"; offending samples can simply be destroyed.

At one recent European meet, according to an official at the scene, a Soviet long jumper and an American thrower both tested positive on their "A" samples. Before their "B" samples could confirm the positives, the meet director walked into the doping control room, picked up the "B" samples, and smashed them on the floor with a dramatic "Whoops!" Which brings us back to the $25-million question: Why didn't someone do the same for Ben?

I would propose two broad possibilities. The first is that no one at Seoul was willing to engage in such damage control on Ben's behalf, despite the looming scandal should Ben's positive become official. The second possibility is that someone *might* have been willing to protect Ben if granted the opportunity, but never got the chance. In that case, we are left with one final puzzle: What might have precluded the rescue of Ben Johnson?

The lab that worked too well. At the crucial juncture when Ben's positive surfaced, conscientious lab personnel proceeded to speed their report of the test results on to the full IOC Medical Commission—before anyone had the opportunity to stop them.

The fatal disclosure. If someone within the lab wanted to remove Ben from the competitive picture, it would make sense to leak the results of his "A" sample *before* the "B" sample was tested—locking the media on to the story.

The Bulgarian pre-empt. According to one tale I was told after Seoul, a Bulgarian doctor happened to drop by the lab just as Ben's name was matched to his positive "A" sample. Still miffed that two weightlifters from his own nation had lost medals after positive tests, the doctor eliminated any chance for Ben to get special treatment—by threatening to blow the whistle if he did.

After Seoul

In the two years that followed the Seoul Olympics, a series of drug-related accusations, confessions, and disclosures rocked track and field. Some were after-shocks of what had happened to Ben, as frantic federations attempted to isolate confessed drug users and protect those who remained in the sport. Other revelations cropped up like bills past due. The conspiracy of silence, the glue that had held the sport together for so many years, was showing its age.

In February 1989, at the U.S.A. Mobil Indoor Track and Field Championships in New York, pole vaulter Billy Olson and shot-putter Augie Wolf both tested positive for testosterone. Don Catlin, the director of the UCLA laboratory which conducted the tests, reported his findings to The Athletics Congress and—in apparent distrust of the national federation—to the IAAF as well. According to an inside source, each sample was tested three times, and each test confirmed the positives. Since Wolf (who has since retired) had been previously suspended for refusing to take a drug test, he would have drawn an automatic lifetime ban had TAC upheld his positive.

A TAC panel, however, declined to suspend either athlete. In claiming victory, Wolf asserted that the testosterone ratio test "was scientifically indefensible." Edwin Moses, a long-time critic of

TAC leader Ollan Cassell, complained that the organization had given its panel inadequate information to overcome the athletes' biochemical defences.

The two reprieves illustrated the arbitrary nature of testosterone testing. While ratios over 6:1 are grounds for automatic suspension at the Olympic Games, IAAF rules allow for "interpretation" at other national and international meets. In explaining why no action was taken against Wolf or Olson, Bob Bowman, a member of TAC's National Athletics Board of Review, hinted at just how far the rules might be bent: "Research has shown that some normal people may have a *75:1 ratio*." (Emphasis added.) Bowman also noted that Wolf and Olson had "tested negative many, many times. We were looking for a trend. One positive test in a string of negatives is important to take into account."

Bowman had turned the two cases on their head. In reality, an athlete with a naturally high testosterone ratio would test positive consistently—as recently confirmed to me by lab director Catlin. One or two isolated positives, on the other hand, would point strongly to an *artificial* altering of the ratio.

It was not the first time that TAC had looked the other way after a positive test, as suggested by a July 18, 1987, letter from George Miller, executive director of the United States Olympic Committee, to Ollan Cassell, his counterpart at TAC. Two days earlier, Miller noted, UCLA's Catlin had telephoned him with news that three athletes' "A" samples had tested positive at the Mobil National Championships in San Jose, California: one for a banned stimulant; a second for the steroid Deca-Durabolin; and a third for a testosterone ratio exceeding 6:1. In addition, Miller reported, eight other samples revealed depressed endocrine profiles, which he ascribed to past steroid use. (The latter group had failed the same test used to disqualify Ben; it is noteworthy that none of these cases was pursued.)

Miller directed Cassell to use his master code to identify the three people with outright positives and to proceed in accordance with protocol. Cassell's next step was to notify the three athletes involved so that they or their agents might be present when their

"B" samples were identified and tested—a formality which almost invariably confirms a positive "A" sample.

We don't know how far Cassell followed his protocol, but we do know this: Not a single athlete was penalized—or even publicly reported as testing positive—after the 1987 national championships in San Jose.

At a December 1988 TAC convention in Phoenix, Cassell laid bare his prime concern about doping: that the embarrassment of positive tests could jeopardize track's future in the United States.

TAC's top official expressed confidence that the state of track and field would improve as a result of a live-coverage contract signed with Turner Broadcasting System, according to minutes recorded by a Nike representative at the convention. "The main stumbling block," the minutes read, "may be a potential scandal involving American athletes, which could be devastating to everyone concerned in America. Canada is presently experiencing such a problem, with practically no interest or support for track."

In this post-Seoul hysteria over the repercussions of drug testing, is it any wonder that Wolf and Olson—and, one might speculate, other American athletes whose names we will never know—were exonerated by TAC? In June 1990, a *Los Angeles Times* investigation, relying on other confidential documents, concluded that TAC officials circumvented their own by-laws when convenient, pressured their drug appeals committee to overturn one case that might have led to a lawsuit, and in some cases simply "forgot" about reported drug positives. In one example, the *Times* reported, Ollan Cassell voided two positives for ephedrine after noting that the low levels involved suggested inadvertent use of the drug—a clear violation of TAC's own rules, which stipulate that the smallest trace of ephedrine dictates a positive test result.

There came a point, however, when even Cassell and his colleagues were forced to act. In April 1989, appearing before the U.S. Senate Judiciary Committee Hearing on Steroid Abuse in America, two-time Olympic sprinter Diane Williams said that her coach, Chuck DeBus, had supplied her with steroids from 1981 to 1984. Williams also testified that positive tests had been concealed at the

U.S. Olympic trials in Los Angeles in 1984, and that she was one of those who escaped. (In commenting on Williams' case, the USOC reported that the "B" sample somehow tested negative after an "A" sample tested positive.)

In September 1989, after IOC president Juan Antonio Samaranch called for the strongest possible penalties for coaches providing banned drugs to their athletes, The Athletics Congress accepted DeBus's two-year "voluntary resignation" from the sport. The *nolo contendere* made both sides happy. Under the written terms of the agreement, DeBus's departure "shall not be deemed an admission of any wrong doing." The arrangement also enabled TAC, which had already collected damaging statements from "eight or nine" athletes, to cancel a dangerous hearing on the case. The deal was later torpedoed, however, by a group of TAC athlete representatives led by Edwin Moses and Harvey Glance. In July 1990, TAC suspended DeBus from the sport for life.

Nor was all quiet on the Eastern front, where long-hidden practices were blown open by *glasnost* and a gathering resentment of elite athletes' wealth and privilege. In addition to *Zmena*'s disclosure about the U.S.S.R.'s floating laboratory at the Montreal Olympics, there were the unequivocal assertions of Sergey Waitchekovsky, the Soviets' head swim coach until 1981. Waitchekovsky maintained that "all" of his athletes had used steroids from 1974 on, in large doses of 50 to 100 milligrams per day. Unlike the East Germans, the coach bragged, his swimmers continued taking the banned substances to within a month of major meets. "I'm an expert and I fixed them all up personally," he explained. "Skillfully administered, drugs need never be discovered." Over eight years the coach slipped only once, when Viktor Kuznetsov tested positive at the 1977 World Cup in Dusseldorf. But even that story ended happily; Kuznetsov went on to win two silver medals at the 1980 Moscow Olympics.

There was also the tale of Igor Larionov, the former Soviet hockey star who now plays for the National Hockey League's Vancouver Canucks. In his book *The Front Line Rebels*, Larionov revealed that some of his teammates passed drug tests at the 1986 World Championships in Moscow by using containers of clean urine that had been hidden behind the toilet bowls at the doping control centre.

(At the European Championships of the same year in Stuttgart, according to Bernd Heller's testimony at the Dubin Inquiry, about 25 percent of the Soviet Union's athletes were pulled from the team at the last moment and stayed home—a suspicious epidemic, in light of *Zmena*'s revelation of the Soviets' rigorous pre-testing practices.)

The earlier reports about steroid use in the G.D.R., meanwhile, were confirmed by a more celebrated defector, Hans-Georg Aschenbach, the former East German ski-jumping champion and 1976 Olympic gold medallist. Elite athletes in the G.D.R. were "forced" to take steroids from adolescence on, he told a West German newspaper: "I swallowed and injected anabolics for eight years."

After the IAAF's John Holt attempted to dismiss such revelations as politically motivated, Aschenbach was seconded in February 1990 by two prominent East German sports scientists who had remained in their country. Top G.D.R. athletes "have been doping here to boost their training for years," said Hermann Buhl, deputy head of medical research at the Leipzig Research Institute for Physical Culture and Sport. "We did research on the dosage and modification of [performance-enhancing] substances....We were the ones whose job was to find the right moment in training when something had to be given." (In the March 1990 issue of the West German magazine *Der Spiegel*, two top G.D.R. officials revealed that their doping research program had enlisted 18 professors, 24 assistant professors, 132 doctors, and 240 other staff people.) To help fine-tune their protocols, the G.D.R. officials used an internal, "off-season" drug testing program. In 1988, as documented in the Dubin report, 23 percent of the 1,400 tests came up positive, yet not a single athlete was referred to the IAAF for possible sanctions.

In a *Toronto Star* story published in June, Buhl amplified his comments, echoing many of the points I made at the Dubin Inquiry a year earlier. Buhl stressed that there was no "wonder drug" in sport. While acknowledging that drugs were essential to modern training demands, he maintained that the G.D.R.'s edge lay not in chemistry, but in coaching and training techniques. He stressed that the East German athletes excelled on *lower* doses of steroids than their Western counterparts; the G.D.R. focused on stringently supervised protocols, rather than high pharmaceutical technology.

Buhl was backed up by an unlikely source—Manfred Donike of the IOC-accredited lab in Cologne. As he told Anne-Lise Hammer, "The Russians know a few drugs, the East Germans are much more sophisticated, but the Americans are the world champions of doping."

As one of the ruling powers of international track, the U.S. long enjoyed laissez-faire governance from the IAAF as long as it gave lip-service to the ideals of drug-free sport. But in the wake of Seoul and various steroid-related brush fires, the Americans were pushed to join the move toward random testing. In October 1989, the U.S. Olympic Committee adopted year-round, out-of-competition drug-testing regulations, to be implemented by TAC. From a pool of the top 15 athletes in each event, a total of 14 randomly selected people would be tested each week.

From the start, however, the program was far less than advertised. Citing a shortage of trained personnel, TAC chopped the program from 52 to 13 weeks per year and announced it would exempt any athlete who lived or trained more than 75 miles from the nearest testing site. In the program's early stages, 175 of the 294 athletes called to be tested—well over half—were excused because they were outside the 75-mile radius. Although Ollan Cassell continually vowed that loophole would be closed, his promises wore thin. In May 1990, four members of TAC's drug-testing committee—including chairman Edwin Moses—resigned in frustration.

"We lost faith" in TAC officials, Moses said. "You just can't believe anything they say."

In resigning, the four athletes followed the lead of Dr. Robert Voy, chief medical officer for the USOC, who'd stepped down from *his* position in the summer of 1989. Shortly before the 1988 Olympics, Voy had created a stir by revealing that there had been positive tests at the U.S. Olympic trials in Indianapolis—an acute embarrassment, as no positives had been announced. After the doctor resigned, he made no secret of his disenchantment. In particular, he complained to the *Los Angeles Times* of rampant ephedrine abuse among sprinters and jumpers. (Ephedrine, a stimulant found in some over-the-counter cold medications, is widely used in much higher concentrations to enhance performance.) "I don't feel that there's a commitment in sports to stop drug abuse," he told the BBC, "because sport...requires contributions by sponsors to support athletes in the program, and unless you win medals and set records, you're not going to get that kind of support.... It's become a great incentive—not only for athletes to do whatever is necessary to gain the competitive edge, but for sports to look the other way when it comes to performance-enhancing substances."

(In his recently published book, *Drugs, Sport, and Politics*, Voy went even further, accusing TAC and the IAAF of cover-ups on the drug issue, and charging that some American athletes have been warned in advance about TAC's random tests. As Voy wrote, "This sport [track and field] has what I believe to be the darkest history when it comes to drug abuse among athletes—and the unwillingness of officials to work effectively toward eliminating" the problem.)

Voy had come to the crux of the matter. International track and field has become a big business—and as in any big business, the bottom line rules. It is no longer enough to "do your best." Through the 1960s, as Canadian writer Varda Burstyn has noted, national sports associations were largely voluntary affairs. The sponsors which funded their Olympic efforts sought prestige more than raw profit. But by the 1970s, as the television audience burgeoned and the Games swallowed more and more air time, and as the extravaganza became ever more costly to produce, the IOC sought closer commercial links with major corporations. Its national constituents (including the U.S. Olympic Committee and, to a lesser degree, the Canadian Olympic Association) followed suit. The federations profited not merely from the handsome sums reeled in for televised commercial spots, but also for the countless spinoffs involving the Olympic five-ring logo. (Leading up to the Winter Olympics in Calgary in 1988, the Canadian Olympic Association sued numerous small businesses to preserve its logo copyright.)

In 1984, ABC paid a then unheard-of $225 million for the 1984 Olympics in Los Angeles, a Games so corporatized that it came to be known as the McLympics. NBC topped its rivals with a $300 million bid for Seoul and $401 million for the 1992 Olympics in Barcelona. These royal sums have become the life's blood of modern track and field—not only for the mounting of the Games themselves, but to support the featherbedding officials who enjoy first-class air travel and plush hotels in exotic places.

Since the networks and their sponsors pay the piper, they expect to call the tune. They demand wholesome (read: drug-free) family entertainment to keep the vast Olympic viewing public content and sheltered from disillusionment. At the same time, they need new world records and superb (read: drug-dependent) performances to keep that public coming back for more.

These conflicting demands sow fertile ground for compromise and caprice. When the IOC's Medical Commission disqualified 10 people at Seoul but opted *not* to act on 20 other positive tests, it subjectively decided who would be lionized and who would be destroyed.

The Fraternity

At the IOC's inner circle sits the Subcommission on Doping and Biochemistry of Sport: Manfred Donike and Claus Clausnitzer of Germany, Arnold Beckett of Britain, Donald Catlin of the U.S., Robert Dugal of Canada, and Vitaly Semenov of the Soviet Union. They certify their own labs and charge all that the market will bear. In 1984, for example, Dugal of Montreal signed a four-year contract with Sport Canada that eventually paid him $400 per urinalysis. During the same period, he accepted a take-it-or-leave-it offer from the National Collegiate Athletic Association of only $185 (U.S.) per test. When the Sport Canada contract came up for renewal in 1988, the inner circle decertified Dugal's only competition, the recently established lab at the Foothills Hospital in Calgary.

Explaining the lab's decision to stop its futile reaccreditation attempts, Dr. Robert Baynton wrote to Donike on November 3, 1989: "In conclusion, this last reaccreditation attempt by our laboratory confirms suspicions that we have had for quite some time—there is no intention by you to reaccredit [sic] this laboratory. If every IOC laboratory was subjected to the same scrutiny and treated as unfairly as us, chances are the number of IOC labs would only number five (5)—exactly the number of members of the subcommission

289

who are heads of IOC laboratories. We know of few other systems where vested interests control and adjudicate so directly."

Ralph Coombs, the president of Foothills Hospital, registered the same disgust in a letter to Donike dated December 20, 1989. "The structure of the subcommission," he wrote, "which permits your members to be the professionals who act as consultants, then accreditors, subsequently adjudicators, and also the appeal group, while maintaining a monopoly commercial interest, defies common standards of public accountability."

If the subcommission's structure enforces an unhealthy monopoly of the urinalysis business in Canada, the inner circle's stranglehold on drug-testing research is likewise sheltered from outsiders. Its work fails to meet the standard for all legitimate science, since it is unpublished and therefore hidden from peer review. Where no one is accountable, lines are drawn arbitrarily. A given urinalysis reading is positive because the lab directors say so.

Yet for all of its unchallenged authority, the "science" behind IAAF drug testing is so tenuous that it provokes disputes even within the fraternity. Donike has emerged as the J. Edgar Hoover of dope busters, the one who pushed hardest for adoption of the testosterone ratio—against the public reservations of Beckett and Dugal that the test was not yet reliable enough for use. A similar battle is materializing over the use of endocrine profiles. Several months after this controversial test was trotted out to snare Ben, Beckett advised *against* its use by the International Weightlifting Federation.

For all their doubts, however, the lab directors continue to rely on these tests, just as they reject athlete appeals out of hand. Their *modus operandi* flies in the face of their public pronouncements: that the majority of athletes are clean. They deny due process because they know the athletes are guilty. They know what it takes to play the game.

The inner circle's dual role—as both subcommissioners and lab directors—undercuts the credibility of their test results. As Dr. Robert Voy told *The New York Times*, "You can't have a sport test itself and be trustworthy. It's like the fox guarding the henhouse."

To compound their clout, the subcommissioners—and their labs—serve both the IAAF and the IOC. (Both Donike and Beckett are also members of the IAAF Doping Commission.) This interlocking directorate belies the claims of IOC vice-president Richard Pound that drug testing is more rigorous in the Olympics than in the IAAF-run World Championships. While there were no official positives in Helsinki and only one in Rome, the dope busters were hardly more prolific in Seoul. In the 1988 Olympics, Ben Johnson represented the single positive in track and field, the only fair standard of comparison. (Since 1968, when the IOC initiated drug testing at the Olympics, it has recorded a *total* of six positives in track and field—an average of one per Games.) The same IOC inner circle is in charge of both the World Championships and the Olympics. It can be no surprise that the results are so similar.

Even now, as the IAAF seeks to assert itself, it can still be foiled by a protective national federation. In 1989, Ljungqvist arrived at the site of the Czech national championships to supervise a drug-testing operation—only to find that the Czechs had already folded their tents, after quietly shifting their biggest meet of the year to one week earlier.

Athletes are no better or worse than the societies from which they come. Their nations clamour for glory. Their sponsors reward success. They are expected to win and yet remain drug-free—goals that have become increasingly incompatible over the last 20 years.

In today's international sport, the pressures are overwhelming. In 1964, an Olympic gold medal might have been a nice piece of memorabilia. Today that medal can be worth millions—and the route to the winner's podium passes through the tablet or syringe.

Even as Sport Canada bathes its athletes in anti-drug rhetoric, it endorses drug-inflated selection and carding standards. (In fact, Sport Canada would have a hard time adjusting its standards even if it wanted to. After decades of steroid-linked performances, no one knows what "clean" performers can do.) When my athletes made their decision to use steroids, they followed the old circuit motto: *If you don't take it, you won't make it.* As Tony Sharpe told the

Dubin Inquiry, "The glory is too sweet, the dollars are too much." Or as shot-putter Augie Wolf put it: "The pressure to take drugs is enormous. An athlete asks himself, 'Do I take drugs and win medals, or do I play fair and finish last?' "

There have always been athletes who were willing to forgo drugs. But these abstainers are unlikely to stop at a single compromise. They tend to be the same people who are unwilling to leave a school or job for full-time training, or to move away from friends and family to find the best possible coach, or to make the myriad other sacrifices that go into becoming a world-class athlete. They may be healthier, more well-rounded individuals for their concessions, but they will not reach the top. The best athletes, for better or worse, are the most single-minded ones.

After Seoul, the advent of random testing in North America—and the general panic atmosphere—was a temporary deterrent for some, as reflected by a dip in performance levels. As Edwin Moses observed, "Times are up and people are skinnier." More recently, the IOC's Samaranch acknowledged that performances at the 1992 Olympics in Barcelona might "not be so good as before" because of the "fight against doping"—a telling concession as to the pervasive state of drug use among elite athletes in the past.

In April 1990, two prominent Americans—long jumper Larry Myricks and hurdler Greg Foster—drew three-month suspensions after testing positive for ephedrine. But these are the rare exceptions. The same money still talks, the same officials run the labs, the same political fear and favour still rule the results. In such a milieu, random testing will be no more effective than meet testing.

The CTFA's random-testing program has had its own credibility problems. In January 1990, doping control officials travelled halfway around the globe to test Canadian athletes in Australia, a week before the Commonwealth Games. But the tests were useless: too close to the meet to snare steroid users, and too late to serve as an anti-embarrassment program, since the results wouldn't be known until after the Games. Closer to home, officials were less energetic. In June, they went to test Ben Johnson for the fourth time since Seoul, in an effort to make sure Ben remained "clean" before his readmission to the sport. To fulfill their quota, the officials needed a second athlete. They settled for the nearest warm body: a friend of Ben's who doesn't even compete.

In a domain where truth has unpleasant consequences, superstars must bow to hypocrisy. As spokespeople for both the sport and their sponsors, they are expected to condemn drug use. The biggest names recite the "Except for Me" chorus. They all agree that drug use is rife—that just about everyone is doing it, "except for me." We can draw one of two conclusions: If all the active athletes who say they're clean *are* clean, then there are no drugs in sport. But if there is a widespread drug problem, as recent developments have made clear, a lot of people are lying.

In Canada, a nation stripped of its true superstar, the whitest hat is worn by Dave Steen, the decathlete who won the bronze medal at Seoul. To redeem their sullied program, Sport Canada and the CTFA were desperate to trot out a drug-free hero, and Steen fit the bill—"an athletic version of Mother Teresa," wrote Peter Worthington in *The Ottawa Sun*. In his own public statements, Steen projected the firmest of anti-drug convictions, though he tempered them with generosity for those weaker than himself. "Many people say that it's Ben's fault, or the fault of the people immediately around him," Steen told journalist Varda Burstyn. "But if they look a little deeper, they'll see that it's society and its values that are also at fault. We've lost the original ethics and morals of sport."

At the Dubin Inquiry, Steen presented an undated letter to the CTFA, said to be written in early 1988, in which he asked to be drug-tested regularly for the rest of his career. During the period before Seoul, however, Steen's place in the anti-drug vanguard was not so clear to those around him. In the agreement he signed with the CTFA for 1988, he crossed out the clause that obliges signers to submit to random, out-of-competition testing. In his testimony, Steen said he'd deleted this provision because he was a member of the CTFA's athletes' advisory council and "felt responsibility to act on behalf of other athletes along with myself." The CTFA lacked enough money to do the job right, he continued, and "didn't know exactly what direction they were heading in.... It was too vague."

But Optimist sprinter Molly Killingbeck told columnist Worthington that the athletes' council had taken no position on the clause, and that Steen had scratched it out on his own. (Molly later advised me that Steen had weighed in with the council majority that opposed random testing.) At no point, she added, did she hear Steen refer to his letter volunteering him for drug tests.

The Future

More than one hundred substances are now banned by the IOC and its constituent groups, and drug-testing technology has become more sophisticated than ever. Gas chromatography can detect a given substance in concentrations as low as five parts per billion. Mass spectrometry then bombards the suspect molecules and splits them into pieces, producing a graph of components—a chemical fingerprint—which is matched by a computer data bank to graphs of known substances.

But for all their bells and whistles, the dope busters remain a giant step behind the dope-users. As Dr. Robert Voy told *The New York Times* after Seoul, "The athletes are ahead of us and have stuff we don't even know about.... Our testing over the last four years has simply not solved the problem."

There are thousands of possible synthetic permutations of the testosterone molecule. The great majority of these steroids remain an unexplored frontier, unknown to both sides of the dope war. If prompted by market forces (that is, by users' demand), private laboratories stand ready to synthesize any number of these steroids—and keep the athletes ahead of the game. Even if a doping control computer flags the steroid as a foreign substance, it will not be able to identify it. Without identification, there can be no official positive.

The louder the track federations preach disarmament, the greater the proliferation of pharmaceutical weapons. For all the attention given to steroids, far more dangerous substances are now being used, many of them beyond the sport's control. Some elite athletes are resorting to insulin, which stimulates protein synthesis in muscles at the risk of self-induced diabetes; human chorionic gonadotropin, a hormone which is extracted from the urine of pregnant women and increases testosterone levels in men; sydnocarb, a "super-amphetamine" several times stronger than Methedrine; and even nerve gas and that old standby, strychnine, both stimulants in small quantities but lethal in overdose. In the spring of 1990, the latest weapon was unveiled: a nationally advertised masking agent called DEFEND. Put out by Power Distributors of Marina Del Rey, California, the product, according to its promoters, "is pleasant tasting, works in less than two hours, and is effective up to five hours. You simply mix with water and drink.

"DEFEND is the ultimate defense weapon against unconstitutional urinalysis testing!

"DEFEND successfully eliminates the detection of metabolites in your urine that could trigger a positive test result!

"DEFEND has...been successfully tested with the oral anabolic steroids such as Anavar and Anadrol 50.

"Armed with the proper knowledge and DEFEND, you can successfully pass an IOC...urinalysis designed to detect performance enhancing substances!"

Steroids have been attacked, first and foremost, as an unacceptable health risk. But while any drug can be abused, and all drugs have side effects, the evidence against steroids is almost wholly anecdotal. The most publicized and frightening allegation—the purported link between steroid use and liver cancer—simply lacks foundation. From 1971 to date, the medical literature contains only two reports of malignant liver tumours among otherwise healthy athletes on steroids. Both of the victims were taking large daily doses of 100 milligrams or more. Neither individual had been studied before the onset of the cancer. And neither report addressed other variables, such as family history or the possibility of some other underlying disorder.

While less serious liver damage has been observed among athletes on steroids, the organ consistently returns to normal after the drugs are discontinued. In addition, athletes who encounter problems may switch from steroids that are *hepatotoxic*, or harmful to the liver (such as Dianabol, Anadrol-50, and Winstrol) to others that are not (Primobolan, Deca-Durabolin, and testosterone, among others). And despite scare stories to the contrary, the connection between steroids and heart disease is more tenuous still, with no documentation in the literature. (Although there is stronger evidence that steroids may contribute to elevated serum cholesterol levels in athletes, the condition can usually be controlled with a combination of diet, bran, and niacin supplements.) When a prominent anti-steroid doctor declared in the days after Seoul that "young athletes who take heavy doses of anabolic steroids for 60 to 90 days should expect to die in their 30s and 40s," he was sounding the sort of alarm that has led generations of steroid users to discount *all* warnings about drugs, whether founded or not.

Rigorous, controlled studies—those comparing populations of steroid users and non-users—have yet to be done, even with lower primates. There is little funding for such research, as mainstream medicine has been content to label these drugs as a problem to be controlled, rather than an issue to be explored. Moral outrage has short-circuited the scientific method.

If the IOC and IAAF drug policies were designed to protect the athletes' health, they have failed. Rather than inducing people to perform without drugs, the banned list has pushed them up the endocrine ladder, to new substances with harsher side effects or unknown risks. In this context, the demonization of steroids has done no one a favour. While hard research remains scanty, what we do know suggests that any adverse effects of commercially marketed steroids are minor and mostly reversible, *as long as dosages are kept low and durations are limited*. The same cannot be said with any confidence of sydnocarb or Pirvitan. Unfortunately, today's athlete is forced to seek not the safest effective drugs, but the ones that are least detectable.

The IAAF has done no better in its second stated mission—to safeguard the fairness and integrity of the sport. In fact, the playing field grows less level by the day. Each advance in testing lends a greater advantage to nations with the technological know-how to keep beating the testers—and the clout to protect their top stars if anything goes wrong. With the right contacts and enough money, athletes in the United States, Italy, or Germany can gain regular access to a lab with the latest equipment. They can beat any testosterone ratio test by injecting epitestosterone along with testosterone during training, and monitoring the results with absolute secrecy within the private lab. While benefiting from a higher testosterone level, these athletes keep their ratios well below the 6:1 threshold. And the IAAF has no way to catch them.

At the Winter Olympics in Calgary in 1988, a new star emerged—not because he was good, but because he was bad. Unbelievably bad. He was a myopic British house painter and part-time ski jumper known as "Eddie the Eagle." Like the Jamaican bobsled team, he served as comic relief for the Games.

In Canada the Eagle has landed. Since we can no longer expect to generate superstars like Ben Johnson, we must content ourselves with participation for its own sake. By the time of the Commonwealth Games in January 1990, sport minister Jean Charest had retreated far from the heady goals of *Toward 2000*. Don't worry about the medal count, he told our team—and be sure to get in some sightseeing.

The "High Performance" insignias on national team uniforms have been replaced with a new motto: "Fair Play." Sport Canada's latest appendage, the Commission for Fair Play, has raised more than $2.6 million for magazine ads and other just-say-no promotions—money that might have helped our underfunded athletes. The officials are sending a message: It's okay to lose, as long as you don't embarrass us.

The message has found its mark. In 1989, the number of Canada's A-carded athletes—those who can compete at an Olympic finalist level—dropped by 38 percent, from 103 to 64.

Canada's poor third in the 1990 Commonwealth Games was merely a taste of what lies in store at the 1991 World Championships in Tokyo. An even more costly fiasco looms at the 1994 Commonwealth Games in Victoria, for which the Canadian government has committed $50 million to show the world how far we have fallen.

International sport is moving irrevocably toward a two-tiered athletic society—to prosecute the great mass of uninformed and expendable players, while giving *carte blanche* to a handful of well-connected superstars. Doping control in the 1990s will formalize *limited, beatable testing*—a controlled and selective roulette without the risk of major scandal. The anxious network sugar daddies will be appeased, the record-hungry fans satiated. And if the competitions become over-produced Hollywood farces, with an ever-widening gap between the few authentic contenders and all the rest with no chance, who will be the wiser?

But I believe there is another way—a safer way, a fairer way. We must acknowledge, first, that prohibitions backfire. Doping has been suppressed in modern track and field no better than drinking was stopped during America's Roaring Twenties. Further, I would submit that the resultant dishonesty has done more harm to the sport than the drugs themselves.

Anabolic steroids were banned on the basis of two false rationales—that they offered an unfair advantage, and that they represented a severe and universal danger to athletes' health, regardless of type or dose. Steroids were not banned because they were unethical; they became unethical because they were banned. Or, as Richard Pound told the Dubin Inquiry, "We have a list. We don't have the ethical framework that indicates why testosterone is bad and something else may be good."

In several other sports where steroid use would appear likely, the drugs are not perceived as a problem, simply because they are not banned or tested for. Nor are steroids deemed a mortal danger by the World Health Organization (WHO), which has sponsored international research into a possible male version of the Pill since 1971. The project's goal, according to Dr. C. Alvin Paulsen, a professor of medicine at the University of Washington School of Medicine, is to find a "safe, reversible, and reasonably effective" method of male birth control. In the most recent WHO experiment, 157 men received weekly injections of 200 milligrams of testosterone enanthate (a long-acting compound of the natural male hormone) for 60 to 68 weeks—a total of more than 10,000 milligrams for each individual. (A similar weekly dose, according to Dr. Mauro DiPasquale, the Canadian expert on steroids, might be used by a sprinter seeking anabolic effects.) According to Paulsen, who supervised one of ten groups in the trial, each subject underwent a monthly physical exam and blood work-up. By the end of the study, the researchers had observed only two adverse effects: acne (in a minority of cases), and some weight gain, averaging six pounds, from water retention.

"We know it (testosterone) won't affect the liver, and we know it won't affect the kidneys or serum cholesterol, because we monitored that," Paulsen said. Moreover, the subjects reported no change in their libido or sexual performance. Even the *intended* effect of the drug—a reduction of sperm count—was temporary and reversible; after the injections ceased, the counts returned to their prior levels.

Unfortunately, synthetic steroids have yet to be put to such a clinical test. Since the synthetics are generally less androgenic than testosterone, they might be less likely to cause problems like acne. And as noted earlier, most oral synthetics pose a potential threat to the liver, though this effect varies widely from substance to substance (stanozolol, the steroid used by our group, would appear to fall somewhere in the middle range), and can be monitored to prevent actual damage. Nonetheless, Paulsen's work—both in the latest testosterone experiment and in similar trials over the last 19 years—has led him to conclude that steroids may be "acceptable in terms of safety within prescribed limits," and that side effects depend entirely "on the dosage and type of steroid."

(Growth hormone, the common complement to steroids among athletes, is also being eyed for new therapeutic uses. According to a July 1990 study published in the *New England Journal of Medicine*, researchers found that growth hormone might turn back the biological clock 10 to 20 years. Led by Dr. Daniel Rudman of the Medical College of Wisconsin in Milwaukee, the study found that most of the elderly male subjects lost fat, regained muscle, strengthened backbones, and developed thicker, more youthful skin after injecting themselves three times a week for six months.)

Steroid use has extended far beyond the athletic community. The public is enticed by steroid-enhanced actors, rock stars, models, and body-builders. Millions of young men want to look like the guys that they see in beer commercials and Calvin Klein ads— and they've long stopped buying the old line that "hard work" will get them there. These are the people who support a steroid black market estimated at $500 million in the United States and another $60 million in Canada. They are ill-served by the criminalization of these drugs. As penalties intensify, fewer doctors will risk prescribing steroids, leaving users without monitoring or reliable advice.

(This state of affairs is particularly injurious to the younger people who use steroids, most of them for cosmetic reasons— 262,000 teenagers in the U.S. alone, according to a recent report by the U.S. Department of Health and Human Services inspector general. These adolescents should not take steroids under *any* circumstances, since the drugs may permanently stunt their growth. In the absence of an honest evaluation and a realistic educational campaign, however, there is little to deter them.)

As a coach, my dilemma was intensified by the fact that my athletes came from among the poorest segments of Canadian society. They pursued careers as sprinters not to "build character" but to make a living as professional athletes in a professional sport. To ask them to eschew drugs used by their international competition would have been to ask them to stay poor. In the post-Dubin era,

Canada is telling them: You cannot make money in your chosen profession. You can never set a world record. You are barred from the big leagues.

Thirty-five years ago, following an age-old tradition, John Ziegler sought a safer, more effective alternative to testosterone, and succeeded with Dianabol. Twenty years ago, sports science turned to a search for blame, which culminated in the vilification of Ben Johnson. I believe it is time to shift back.

Our new era would begin to define a different role for sports science, not as a cop on the beat, but as the athletes' partner in expanding the possibilities of human performance. It is time for the IAAF to promote and sponsor its own open, international research on performance-enhancing drugs. We must demystify these substances, and define both their risks and their benefits.

If we are to have drug testing worthy of its name, it must be administered by an independent agency, one without ties to the commercial side of the sport. Of equal importance, the tests themselves must withstand the most exacting scientific scrutiny. They must be reliable, reasonable, and universally applied.

In an ideal world, of course, people would not feel so impelled to seek an edge—pharmaceutical or otherwise—over their competition. Athletes would pursue excellence for its own sake; in such a world there would be little demand for performance-enhancing drugs. But as long as sport remains a big business; as long as the Olympics are driven by the dollar first and last (from the IOC's nine-figure network revenues to the gold medallist's seven-figure commercial endorsements); as long as hundredths of seconds translate into millions of dollars and blinding celebrity, athletes will do whatever they can to win.

But in the real world, there is no ideal solution to the problem of drug use in sport. On a more practical level, however, we could surely improve the current system of testing. If the IAAF were truly concerned about shielding its athletes from the worst hazards of drugs, as opposed to catching the occasional unfortunate, it would drop its banned list altogether. Rather than hunt for trace amounts of specific substances, it would focus upon the *general* impact of drug use on each athlete's health. To that end, the independent testing agency might develop an endocrine profile—a set of hormone ratios—that would be far more sophisticated than either the unproven version invoked against Ben in Seoul or the crude testosterone/epitestosterone test with its problematic 6:1 threshold.

Technologically, this development is within our sights. The testesterone ratio test, for example, could be made far more reliable if supplemented by ratios involving other substances, including luteinizing hormone, which is produced by the pituitary gland and which regulates testosterone production in men.

The philosophy behind this approach is simple. If athletes are doped to the point where their own hormonal production is significantly disrupted—regardless of the particular drug or drugs involved—they are more likely at risk, and should be reined in. A first offence might call for a three-month suspension, a second offence for one year, a third offence for two years or more. The emphasis, however, would be on *protecting* the athletes, not punishing them.

In the same spirit, the endocrine profile would be packaged with regular blood work-ups to monitor the three leading risk areas for steroid users: liver function, kidney function, and cholesterol levels. These tests would be wholly non-punitive.

I would be the first to concede that the endocrine profile is an imperfect guardian. As with any test, an arbitrary line would have to be drawn between acceptable and unacceptable variations in endogenous (natural) hormone levels. And although an endocrine profile would be harder to manipulate than tests for specific steroids, the more enterprising and privileged athletes would inevitably find a way.

As I envision it, the profile would be a check against dangerous drug abuse, rather than a tool to stamp out any and all use of performance-enhancing substances. It will not satisfy the prohibitionists. But the profile's limitation might turn out to be a virtue; like most complex problems, the issue of drugs in sport is better addressed by honest (if partial) measures than by sweeping moral campaigns.

Steroids are potent drugs. They require carefully planned protocols and the direct supervision of a qualified physician. But if mature and informed elite athletes conclude that they must take steroids to survive in their sport, and can do so without jeopardizing their health, they should be able to make that choice freely— and without the lying and hypocrisy which have so damaged track and field.

We allow our elite athletes to engage in boxing and downhill skiing, sports where the documented incidence of serious injury or death is far greater than for a track star taking Dianabol or Winstrol. We permit adolescent girls to attempt dangerous manœuvres like "the Yurchenko," a backward launch onto the vaulting horse (which landed one American in a coma at the Tokyo World Sports Fair in 1988), or to arch their backs to the point where they grind down—and permanently deform—soft, young vertebrae. There is no official outcry against these demonstrated health hazards. They are deemed part of the athletic territory, a crowd-pleasing ingredient of the show. But steroids are treated differently—not because we know them to be more dangerous, but because political fashion and a powerful lobby of lab directors have pushed for a crackdown.

Even people who grant this argument, however, might object to chemical interference into what they consider a "natural" endeavour. I would counter that we ceased being natural ages ago, the moment we stopped running barefoot on dirt paths. It is a formidable challenge to distinguish between nature and artifice, a task I would leave to philosophers.

But I was a sprint coach, and I had a different job: to help a few gifted people run as fast as they could.

Coda

Two years after Seoul, the people who forged Canada's greatest sprint team are still sorting out their lives. In late 1989, the Ontario Provincial Police charged Ross Earl, the most selfless man I ever met, with violating the terms of the Scarborough Optimist bingo licence. (The charges involved such high crimes as advancing rent money to Angella Issajenko, whose carding allowance was paid erratically, and buying a wedding gift for an Optimist high-jump coach who'd given 15 years to the club. In June 1990, all charges against Ross and three other club directors were dropped.) No longer active in track and field, Ross now coaches youth volleyball.

Gerard Mach, squeezed out of his job after the Olympics, suffers from heart trouble and is making do with a small CTFA pension.

Jamie Astaphan is practising medicine in St. Kitts. In June 1990, he was charged with professional misconduct by the College of Physicians and Surgeons of Ontario in connection with his administration of steroids to Canadian athletes. If the charges are upheld in a hearing scheduled for June 1991, he could lose his licence to practise in Ontario and be fined up to $10,000.

Waldemar Matuszewski's contract was not renewed by the CTFA. He is currently living in Ottawa.

Angella Issajenko had her second daughter in November of 1989 and has retired from competition. Her recently published autobiography, *Running Risks*, offers a frank account of her own experience with performance-enhancing drugs.

Tony Sharpe has also retired, and is selling cars in Toronto.

Desai Williams is attempting a comeback, working on his own.

Mark McKoy has been shuttling between Toronto and Wales, where he is training with British high-hurdles record-holder Colin Jackson.

In January 1990, sport minister Jean Charest resigned after it became public that he had phoned a judge presiding over a case that involved the CTFA.

In March 1990, Charles Dubin was named Chief Justice of Ontario.

In the spring of 1990, the CTFA adopted a new name: Athletics Canada. Its leadership and policies, however, remain unchanged.

In August, Sport Canada stiffened its first-offence penalty for a positive steroid test to a four-year suspension—the heaviest sanction in the world. As acknowledged by Dick Pound, the IOC vice-president, this amounts to "a death penalty" for professional athletes, given their brief careers.

As this book went to press, Ben Johnson was preparing to return to the sport with a full schedule of competitions in 1991. "I want to take back the titles and the records I have been deprived of," he announced, shortly before his two-year IAAF suspension expired on September 24, 1990. During the months before his return, Ben trained for a time with my old mentor, Percy Duncan (now 75 years old), and brought Super Mike back to Toronto as his personal masseur.

On September 28, 1990, the Canadian Olympic Association completed Johnson's reinstatement by announcing that he would be allowed to rejoin the Canadian national team and to compete at the Barcelona Olympics in 1992. In the meantime, a big-money showdown with Carl Lewis seems likely.

19207

362.29   Francis, Charlie
FRA
          Speed trap

$18.95

DATE			

001242   433603